As Taylor so truthfully puts it in her authentic and inspiring new book, *Eat the Cookie*, when she says, "Comparison is the thief of joy," she offers women a more beautiful path rooted in Christ himself. What a gift to us all! Women of all walks will be able to relate to her loving and humorous account of her own perfectionistic struggles and the freedom that comes with seeking our identity in our Lord. Plus, who doesn't want fantastic recipes and great workouts to accompany Holy Scripture? Well done, Taylor!

Rose Rea, founder of *Radiant* and *Valiant* magazines,
creator of the coffee-table book *Spirit and Life*

As a recovered bulimic and veteran in ministry to women with disordered eating, I can say with confidence, Taylor Kiser gets it. Her depth of understanding surrounding both the temptations and triggers of disordered thoughts and behaviors when it comes to food and body image, as well as the biblical truths and principals that lead to freedom, are spot on. Taylor is a great communicator: relatable, authentic, and super vulnerable. I'll definitely be recommending *Eat the Cookie* to the women coming through our Eyes Wide Open healing program.

Rae Lynn DeAngelis, author, speaker, founder/
executive director of Living in Truth Ministries

Taylor Kiser's book, *Eat the Cookie*, is like taking in a big breath of fresh air and letting it all out. It's a feeling of relief and freedom to truly be who God created us to be. This book will help heal your heart, no matter who you are, no matter what you've been through—whether you've dealt with insecurities, food rules, or mental battles. Taylor has a gift of feeding people with God's love as well as feeding us with nourishing recipes, yes, even cookies! Because let's be honest, life's too short not to enjoy that sweet goodness.

Lindsay Cotter, gluten-free nutrition specialist,
author of *Nourishing Superfood Bowls*

Eat the Cookie is a beautifully raw and entertaining masterpiece. Taylor has discovered what hundreds are seeking: the secret to freedom and true recovery from disordered eating and thinking. I simply couldn't put it down!

Lindsey Racz, licensed professional counselor, psychology instructor, eating disorder specialist

Taylor's candid journey of her personal battles and victories with food in *Eat the Cookie* is both captivating and transformative. She makes you laugh, feel spiritually lighter, and experience confidence as you walk away not only with biblical knowledge but also with fun new workouts and mouth-watering recipes you can't wait to go try for yourself.

Kasey Shuler, author of *Move for Joy*

In *Eat the Cookie*, Taylor calls us out of the trap of perfection and into the realm of freedom. Rooted in Scripture and full of practical insight, *Eat the Cookie* will make you reconsider your relationship with food and exercise in light of the gospel. Taylor shares her own struggles and triumphs and, with grace and humility, urges readers down a better path. So grab a cookie (or make some of Taylor's), and dig into a life-changing read!

Aubrey Golbek, registered dietitian, author of *Grace, Food, and Everything In Between*

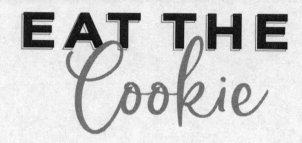

EAT THE *Cookie*

THE IMPERFECTIONIST'S GUIDE TO

FOOD, FAITH, AND FITNESS

Taylor Kiser

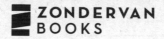

ZONDERVAN BOOKS

ZONDERVAN BOOKS

Eat the Cookie
Copyright © 2020 by Taylor Kiser

Requests for information should be addressed to:
Zondervan, 3900 *Sparks Dr. SE, Grand Rapids, Michigan 49546*

Zondervan titles may be purchased in bulk for educational, business, fundraising, or sales promotional use. For information, please email SpecialMarkets@Zondervan.com.

ISBN 978-0-310-35796-4 (audio)

Library of Congress Cataloging-in-Publication Data

Names: Kiser, Taylor, 1990- author.
Title: Eat the cookie : the imperfectionist's guide to food, faith, and fitness / Taylor Kiser.
Description: Grand Rapids : Zondervan, 2020. | Includes bibliographical references. | Summary: "In Eat the Cookie, fitness coach and popular food blogger Taylor Kiser equips you to be health-conscious yet not calorie-obsessed as she shares spiritual truths, delicious recipes, and practical workout plans that inspire you to give up the comparison game and live as the masterpiece you are"—Provided by publisher.
Identifiers: LCCN 2019057936 (print) | LCCN 2019057937 (ebook) | ISBN 9780310357865 (trade paperback) | ISBN 9780310357957 (ebook)
Subjects: LCSH: Self-perception—Religious aspects—Christianity. | Perfection.
Classification: LCC BV4598.25 .K57 2020 (print) | LCC BV4598.25 (ebook) | DDC 248.4—dc23
LC record available at https://lccn.loc.gov/2019057936
LC ebook record available at https://lccn.loc.gov/2019057937

All Scripture quotations are taken from The Holy Bible, New International Version®, NIV®. Copyright © 1973, 1978, 1984, 2011 by Biblica, Inc.® Used by permission of Zondervan. All rights reserved worldwide. www.Zondervan.com. The "NIV" and "New International Version" are trademarks registered in the United States Patent and Trademark Office by Biblica, Inc.®

This book is written as a source of information only. The information contained in this book should by no means be considered a substitute for the advice of a qualified medical professional, who should always be consulted before beginning any new diet, exercise, or other health program.

All efforts have been made to ensure the accuracy of the information contained in this book as of the date published. The author and the publisher expressly disclaim responsibility for any adverse effects arising from the use or application of the information contained herein.

Any internet addresses (websites, blogs, etc.) and telephone numbers in this book are offered as a resource. They are not intended in any way to be or imply an endorsement by Zondervan, nor does Zondervan vouch for the content of these sites and numbers for the life of this book.

No part of this publication may be reproduced, stored in a retrieval system, or transmitted in any form or by any means—electronic, mechanical, photocopy, recording, or any other—except for brief quotations in printed reviews, without the prior permission of the publisher.

The author is represented by the literary agency of Alive Literary Agency, www.aliveliterary.com.

Cover design: James W. Hall IV
Cover photo: Taylor Kiser
Interior design: Denise Froehlich

Printed in the United States of America

20 21 22 23 24 25 26 27 /LSC/ 16 15 14 13 12 11 10 9 8 7 6 5 4 3 2 1

To my wonderful hubs
Always and forever

CONTENTS

CHAPTER 1

EMBRACE IMPERFECT PERFECTION

Perfection is not attainable, but if
we chase perfection we can catch
excellence.

—Vince Lombardi

Beep, beep, beep went the heart monitor. The one I was
attached to. The one that notified me every time I moved
too quickly and got my heart rate up too high. The one that
warned me every single day that I just might die.

As I lay in my hospital bed—a tiny, frail, and malnourished
thirteen-year-old girl—I was terrified. Just a few months ago I
was excited to be starting high school, making new friends,

having crushes on boys, and entering this new chapter in my life. I didn't picture that it would start out in a yellow room with fake flowers on the wall that were supposed to make me happy. They didn't make me happy. Nothing made me happy.

Not even the teeny tiny, and very sick, body I now lived in. I still thought I had weight to lose.

Man, I really thought visible abs would be the key to my happiness.

"Perfection." The word that makes us all squirm but also kind of makes us feel excited at the same time. We know in our heads that it isn't something we should be striving for because, girlfriend, we both know you and I have a few things to work on. What we know in our hearts to be true is that it's unattainable. But if we're going to sit down over a glass of wine and have a heart-to-heart, I am pretty sure we would all confess that we all want this unattainable thing we call perfection. Badly.

Now, I'm not a gambling sort of gal, but when I sit down and ponder "perfection," I am willing to bet big dollars that it looks different for everyone. Maybe you want the perfect 4.0 GPA. Or maybe it's a perfect house with a picket fence and that standard 2.5 kids. Or maybe perfection to you is waking up, putting on your power suit and Christian Louboutins, jumping in your Mercedes, and going to the office where you are the CEO.

Whatever your idea of perfection is, I bet you have something that you're striving for. Not that having these desires is a bad thing. I am not going to tell you to let your homework slide or to let your kid be crazy, but when that desire becomes absolutely everything in your life and you'll do anything to achieve perfection, that is when it becomes an issue. For many of us, we may not even realize we're chasing after perfection because, on the outside, so many of these goals we have for ourselves look perfectly healthy and like things we should truly be chasing. It's not until we dig way down deep into our souls and get honest with ourselves about the ickiness living there that we realize we're trying to walk the path of perfection. And girlfriend, that's no yellow brick road. That's an ugly, curvy, scary path through the dark forest that no one should be trying to walk.

Spoiler alert: There is hope and freedom and joy in jumping off that scary, dark path. Plus, you'll stop getting nasty cobwebs in your hair.

For me, I struggled with perfection in a lot of ways. Growing up, I always had to have perfect grades. I wanted to have perfect relationships that were a breeze. I dreamed of having the perfect job. But my biggest, most consuming struggle that kept me on that dark, scary pursuit of perfection? That was my struggle with my body, and I'm willing to bet (apparently I *am* a gambling girl) most of you lovely ladies have struggled with this at some point in your life—maybe even right now. Even if you haven't, you know the pressure to be perfect in some area of your life.

When we're talking about our body image, it's so easy to see why we feel suffocated by the pressure to look a certain way. Wherever we go, our eyeballs are bombarded with images of stick-thin, gorgeous models and actresses who look so happy and like they're having the time of their lives. I'm willing to bet (because why not keep going?) that they're not happy. They're *hungry*. But that is beside the point. We assume we must achieve that brand of perfection. These women are perfect. Their bodies are perfect, their lives are perfect, they have some perfect-looking guy, and they probably even look perfect when they're cleaning their bathrooms. Maybe that last one is just me.

We see these images and are so quick to forget one of my very favorite verses. (So favorite that I have part of it tattooed on my arm. I'll show you if we ever hang out, which I hope we do.) Psalm 139:14 says, "I praise you because I am fearfully and wonderfully made; your works are wonderful, I know that full well." It's almost like we read that verse with "media-colored glasses" and assume God isn't talking to *us* in that verse. How could he be when we don't look like, have the same things, or do the same things as the "wonderfully made" women in the media? Maybe he's talking to *those* women, the ones who look "perfect" or are the boss of a big company, or the supermoms who have it all together. But he's definitely not talking to us.

Girlfriend, get your head in the game.

He is talking to *you*.

When I was in my *very* early teen years, these images of beautiful models with "perfect" bodies, long legs, and lean abs brainwashed me, and I fell into the lie that I needed that perfection in my life to be happy, quickly forgetting that God was talking to *me* in Psalm 139:14. I began eating less and exercising more. I lost weight. People complimented my extreme weight loss. I felt *good*. I felt *happy*. Maybe I was becoming like those models on TV!

I was. I was *hungry*.

But I also looked fabulous. So I just kept going, because the biggest lie of chasing perfection is that eventually you will get to a place where you have achieved it, and there will be sunshine and rainbows and unicorns, and you will feel whole and satisfied. But I'm here to call *lies* on perfection, because that just isn't true. I achieved the goal of a model body and still was not satisfied. I kept striving and striving and striving until all that striving and chasing led me to a hospital bed attached to heart monitors, nurses who woke me up in the wee hours of the morning to make sure I was still alive, and a whole lot of hospital food.

If you've ever been in the hospital, you cringed right along with me at the thought of mushy peas and creepy green Jell-O.

However, this was a wake-up call. After five weeks of sitting on my butt in a hospital bed and only having the Bible to get me through, I started to believe what Psalm 139:14 said about me. Maybe I was wonderfully made just as I was. Maybe God was *really, truly* talking to me. Slowly but surely, I grabbed his hand and made my recovery. I asked the doctors for chocolate cake instead of Jell-O because it was scarier, but it made me freer. It was so terrifying at first, but with every meal I asked God to give me the strength to do the next right thing. To eat the next scary food. During this time I truly found my own faith. Not the faith that was instilled in me because I grew up in a Christian home, but the kind of faith where I truly *felt* God's presence. It was a beautiful thing, and it allowed me to walk into wholeness.

I gained the weight back. I got my period back, and I began to feel freedom again. After spending five weeks in the hospital, I had to spend another five months in bed at home, away from school and away from my friends. It was an extremely hard and trying time, but it was also another time when I was able to lean on God and experience him in a way I had never experienced him in the past. It also made me never want to go back to the Perfection Pursuit again.

After I was deemed medically healthy, it was a beautiful seven years of bliss and embracing the parts of me I didn't love but that I knew God had made and designed. I learned how to renew my mind and think about myself the way God thought about me. I spent my days not even remembering what a calorie was. Eating a brownie wasn't even something that would register as scary for me anymore. And I definitely didn't feel the need to jump on a treadmill or pound the pavement to burn it off.

In fact, I even had these brownies I now lovingly call "boy brownies." (See recipe on page 217). They're basically just a brownie recipe loaded with caramel and chocolate chips that I made for all my boyfriends growing up to make them fall in love with me. I hope my husband isn't reading this right now, or he might know that he wasn't the only one who received these! But I ate boy brownies with my boyfriends. I ate non–boy brownies with my girlfriends. I just ate. I exercised healthily. I had a little squish under my belly button, and my thighs no longer had a gap between them. And you know what? I was totally fine with it because I was finally happy. I had experienced the "perfect" body already, and I knew that it led to a pit of despair, and I was *not* crawling back down into that pit again. I no longer felt the weight of perfection. I understood that the Perfection Pursuit was endless and dark and scary and full of icky cobwebs. I was feeling like I was living the best life that God had for me.

Until I wasn't.

One of my favorite verses is John 10:10: "The thief comes only to steal and kill and destroy; I have come that they may have life, and have it to the full." It says that the enemy will use every little trick and lie on us, and not just about how we think about our bodies. Anytime we are pursuing perfection in *any* area of our lives—work, relationships, families, our home—it's the thief coming to steal, kill, and destroy us because he knows that perfection is truly unattainable in any area.

If we fast-forward those seven years to my early twenties, we find the enemy worming his sneaky little self into my life, wanting to steal it, to kill the bliss I was feeling, and to *destroy* me. And you know how he did it? By putting me back on the dark, scary path to perfection. It didn't start as pursing the perfect body. It started with wanting the perfect lifelong relationship. As a single person, I was so desperate to get married. I had my whole wedding planned on Pinterest and was just waiting for the right groom. I thought I had found "the one" and was getting ready to put my Pinterest board into action . . . when we broke up.

That dream died and made me feel completely out of control. I know I'm not the only one who looks to another area of her life to try to control when something else feels out of control, and that is exactly what happened after this breakup. I went back to controlling the one thing I knew how to control— food. I was back at the gym, back obsessing about my body and food and any little thing that went in my mouth. And all that obsessing left no space in my brain to think of God, the one who could take the obsession away.

My body began to change and, yet again, I had the praise of culture and society. I was fit, and everyone thought I looked amazing. I would have never told you then that I was also not sleeping, exhausted, hungry, and angry almost all the time because I just told myself it was "part of the lifestyle." I had the kind of hard-core dedication not to even eat one cookie at Christmas. Girlfriend, have you ever met a person who didn't eat one Christmas cookie? I can tell you from personal experience that you *do not* want to. They are very sad, distressed people who just truly want to *eat that cookie*. I can tell you from experience because I was one of them for a long time.

Doing things perfectly and "having it all together" are praised by our culture, so it was so easy to let it roll off my back and not acknowledge that I was going back down the path of perfection. This struggle isn't only about our bodies, so don't think you're getting off easy if you haven't had that specific struggle. Our culture praises perfection in any category, whether that means becoming the top woman at work or having perfect kids, a perfect house, or a perfect husband. Anytime you feel some kind of worth or value because you "have it all together," no matter what area of life we're talking about, it's going to be a recipe for disaster.

The root of perfection is fear, although you might not know it yet. It could be fear that you will lose your value if you don't have six-pack abs or fear that the world will think you are a failure as a parent if your kid has a temper tantrum, or if you fear, like I used to, that your relationship will never be perfect and therefore you will never be "complete." They're all related to perfection and not wanting the world to think we don't "have it all together." Because who wants to be normal when you can be perfect, right?

Because the enemy knows about our root issue of fear, even if you don't know your specific fear yet, he can use your walk down the Perfection Pursuit against you. For a little while, he won't bug you. I mean, why would he? Anytime you're walking down the Perfection Pursuit, you're already going down a dark path all by yourself. You're making his job easy. He will let you go on your merry little way, holding on to fear and doing everything you can until you feel like you've arrived in your pursuit for body perfection, family perfection, job perfection, or insert any kind of perfection here. You'll feel satisfied. You'll arrive. You'll feel good about what you've done.

Until you don't.

I know women who have spent years crafting the perfect-looking family while still feeling like something was missing. Or women who finally become the CEO of their own company but still feel empty inside. Personally, I spent years working out and eating healthy so that I could get in the best shape of my life. I got there. I was happy for a second. But then I wanted more. I wanted to be pushed more to see if I could get more muscle. I sought the help of a trainer because I figured that would help me get to where I could be, and then I could finally rest knowing that I was enough and had achieved all my goals.

First Peter 5:8 says, "Be alert and of sober mind. Your enemy the devil prowls around like a roaring lion looking for someone to devour," and I was right there ready to be devoured because my mind was not sober or alert. It was focused on achieving, striving, and body perfection. It was too crowded with other thoughts and obsessions to even think about God. Everything that I had learned about being fearfully and wonderfully made and made in the image of God (Genesis 1:26) just flew out of my head, and in came the enemy, read to steal, kill, and destroy.

I'd like to say God has been a part of my life ever since my hospitalization, but if I'm being truly honest with myself, at this point in my life he wasn't there at all. Striving for that "more" and that challenge got me even more fit, sure. But, girlfriend, you know what it also did to me? It made me feel like a crazy person and left me feeling unsatisfied and truly imperfect.

Funny how that works, eh?

Let me just tell you about "purse chicken." Once I was of legal drinking age, I always made sure to have baggies of cooked chicken breast in my purse when my friends and I would head to a bar so that I could sit in a bathroom stall and eat it to avoid eating greasy, fattening bar food. All in the name of trying to achieve that perfect body.

If you ever met a person who ate chicken out of her purse in bathroom stalls to avoid having to eat other foods at parties, or was a really angry person all day if she was going out for dinner with you because she didn't want to eat beforehand to "save calories," or just wouldn't go out for dinner with you *at all* because she only allowed herself to eat her own boring food (probably that nasty purse chicken), would you be her friend?

Probably not. You'd think she was a lunatic.

Hi! I'm Taylor, and that was me.

My own family didn't enjoy spending time with me, and most of the time my husband didn't either. We argued and fought, and I couldn't go on date-nights. My family was concerned about my new lifestyle and weight because they saw all the warning signs happening again that led me down the road to the hospital. But I ignored them.

I told you, chasing perfection made me do a whole bunch of questionable things, like eating food out of baggies and putting tension on my closest relationships. I'm hoping that you've been able to look at some of your own desires as you've been reading along and noticing if you've been pursuing certain aspects of your life for the wrong reasons. Maybe you're able to start to identify some pretty questionable things you have done in hot pursuit of whatever your goal is. Now, remember, goals are great. But white-knuckling onto those goals for dear life and allowing them to take away your worth and value as the beautiful daughter of the King that you are if they don't work out as picture-perfect as you imagined is a problem.

Especially if they lead you to sit in a bathroom stall eating chicken out of your purse.

Worse than crazy Taylor, though, was unsatisfied Taylor, and I'm thinking you're probably really going to identify with this one. There always seemed to be more that I could be doing. More weight to lose, more muscle to gain, more chicken to eat, and so on. I gained more muscle, lost more fat, and I thought it would make me happy and that I would think I finally had that perfect physique that I craved. But that never happened. Literally, not once did I think, "Oh, this is good. I've achieved this perfect body, and now I can just stay here." And this isn't just about bodies. Ever thought, "Oh, my family is finally exactly how I want it"? Or, "I have arrived at the exact job I want, and I will love it every day forever"? Probably not.

Like I said before, the enemy will leave you alone while you carve your own dark path to perfection, until he sees you've reached your goal. Then here comes that roaring lion, holding on to your fear and waving it in your face so that it becomes so scary and real that you forget to be satisfied with how far you have come, and you only want more, more, and *more*. More muscle. Even better grades. A bigger house. More power at work. You name it, and he will tell you that you need it. And once you get it, you'll be left feeling unsatisfied again and feeling like you can just never seem to grasp this perfection thing that everyone else seems to have. The more you feel imperfect, the more the vicious, never-ending cycle continues. The goal is never reached, and the cycle spins on and on.

Sound like you? Don't worry, girlfriend, we're going to band together like a pack of girls with PMS looking for chocolate and overcome that roaring lion with God's *truth*. And we all know that you don't mess with *one* girl craving chocolate, let alone a *pack*. Add in God's truth, and the enemy doesn't have a chance.

No matter how hard we try, we can't be perfect. Our ability to be perfect jumped ship when Adam and Eve bit into the apple in the Garden of Eden. Only God is perfect, and he doesn't want us to be competing with that. But we do. I know I sure did, and it was one of the reasons I was so far from God at this point in my life. When we become obsessed with pursuing perfection, we can only handle one obsession, one pursuit. While I was obsessed with having a perfect body, there was no room for me to pursue God.

However, God isn't telling us, "Oh well, you can never be perfect, so just go do whatever and have no goals." God may not call us to perfection, but he does call us to excellence. They sound similar, but they are much, much different.

To me, the definition of perfection is being totally flawless. You have no defects whatsoever. Of course, trying to get to this level of "flawlessness" usually keeps you stuck in a vicious cycle that never really gets you anywhere. Then, though, there is excellence. To me, excellence is just about being really good, but not perfect, because perfection isn't really possible. No matter how many makeup commercials promise you can achieve flawlessness, it just is not realistic.

In Gretchen Saffles's book *Proverbs 31*, she says, "Perfection looks within ourselves to find joy and happiness, but it always comes up lacking."[1] Excellence still calls you to a life of striving, but in a greater, deeper way. Now we're not striving for perfection, but striving to step into grace and freedom. Gretchen goes on to say, "Excellence looks to Jesus to find wholeness and satisfaction,"[2] and that is because he is the author of that grace and freedom we're now striving for. I just love this perspective. God is the author of excellence, and this is what he wants for you. Joy! Freedom! Satisfaction! Wholeness! Bliss!

You will know when you have arrived at excellence because you will give yourself the grace that God has already given you. When I was on the Perfection Pursuit, there was literally not one iota of grace. If I ate one extra gram of food, I was "bad" and felt ashamed for my lack of willpower and failure as a human. But when I started to shift from the pursuit of perfection to excellence, grace came into play. Grace says that I am human, and that I am going to make mistakes, and that is okay.

Although I now do not think that eating an extra gram of anything should be something to be ashamed of, I did at the time, and grace got me through that. Knowing I was still the same person on the inside and that God still loved me even though I made a "mistake," and allowing myself to move forward with my day is when I knew things had begun to shift. I was starting to make space for a perfect God, because the walk down the Perfection Pursuit of my body was coming to an end.

The Perfection Pursuit does not allow you to make a mistake. When a mistake happens, you will feel it in your very soul. That mistake will crush you. Excellence whispers in your ear, "It's okay. You're doing the best you can, and you are enough. Right here. Right now. Even in the middle of your mess." Learning to listen to that small whisper, actually accepting it to be true, and being okay is how you will be able to pursue excellence in a way that doesn't just end with you walking down the dark and scary Perfection Pursuit once again.

There is no such thing as perfection. Perfection is an

impossible quest—that's the bad news. The good news is we were made to aim for something better and within reach. Realizing our imperfection and beginning to strive for excellence is the only thing we need to focus on.

So what does kicking perfection to the curb and welcoming a life of excellence look like, and how the heck do we get there when the whole wide world is telling us that just being extremely good (whatever that means) isn't good enough? Two things have helped me become a perfection quitter: identifying the difference between the lies and truths in my walk down the dark and scary path of perfection, and then taking up my cross and following Jesus into the freedom and joy that he has for me.

ASK TOUGH QUESTIONS

Don't worry, we're not talking about questions like, Does your handbag need to match your shoes? I don't know about you, but I'm still confused by that one. We're talking about grabbing your shovel and digging *deep* within yourself and asking yourself some hard questions:

1. Why do I feel the need to be perfect in this area?
2. What has striving for this perfection brought to my life?

For me, it wasn't until I truly answered these two questions that I was able to see that this never-ending, vicious cycle wasn't bringing me any kind of joy, I was doing it for all the wrong reasons, and it was truly pulling me away from my most important relationship—the one I had with God. If we were talking at a coffee shop right now, and we were getting into the nitty-gritty with each other, and I had to answer these questions out loud to you, my answers would go something like this:

1. Because if I don't have a perfect body with a visible six-pack and insane leanness, the world will not think I am attractive.
2. Perfect body.

I would then dig down deep into an even scarier, darker part of myself that I would never want to admit really exists, and I would have to unpack why being attractive was so important to me. Would it bring me value or acceptance? And yes, as much as I hate to say these words out loud, I thought it would.

Okay, your turn. Question one. Go deep, go dark, get into the nitty-gritty part of your soul. I'll wait.

I don't know what answers you found, but don't let them make you feel ashamed or guilty. I know I sure did when I unpacked the thought that being attractive would somehow bring me value. Confess that wrong thinking and move on! God held me and loved me through those lackluster, wrong thoughts, which allowed me to move past the feeling of guilt and shame, and I know he will do the same for you. In fact, 1 John 1:9 says that "If we confess our sins, he is faithful and just and will forgive us our sins and purify us from all unrighteousness." The Lord will redeem those thoughts, which will begin to free you to pursue excellence. Remember, excellence is freedom, wholeness, and *joy*!

Okay, question two. This one was the real kicker for me. If you're a list maker (like me), making an old-school list of pros and cons is really helpful. On one side, put "pros of a perfect body," and on the other "cons of a perfect body."

You know what my only pro was? "Perfect body."

Nothing else. Nada. Zipola. Zilch.

The con list was long. It included things like "being hungry," "feeling weak and tired almost all the time," "not sleeping well at night," "having obsessive thoughts about food," "never enjoying date-night because I'm too afraid to eat 'scary food,'" "having no friends because I can't go out for dinner," "nasty, cold purse chicken," "being depressed," "not being the same person I used to be," and "fighting with my husband."

The list went on and on and on and on.

So what has the quest for perfection brought you? I'm willing to bet your list of pros and cons is going to look similar to mine. And if you're anything like me, this list is going to be an eye-opener. Why do we continue chasing something that is bringing us no joy? Even if the media/culture is telling us it will, we have firsthand, personal experience that it does not.

I was never more joyful with less weight or more muscle, but instead I had no friends, no energy, and constant arguments with my husband. I'm sure you're not more joyful when your house is more organized, but you lash out at your kids for finger-painting on the table, risking making a mess of your prized organization, instead of getting right in there and painting with them. The same idea applies to whatever you've been striving for. While you might feel more at peace when your house is organized, it's never worth lashing out at your kids. The feeling that you get after something like that happens is far away from the peace that the clean house brought you in the first place.

TAKE UP THAT CROSS

Now that we've done some soul-searching and list making, and confessed our thoughts about why we have been on this pursuit, it's time to walk into the excellence that God has designed for you. Yes, you! I am not looking at someone else right now. He is ready and waiting with big open arms for you to be okay with being good and not perfect. I know this from experience, because it wasn't until I embraced this concept that I felt God's embrace, truly made space for a perfect God in my life, and was able to reach out and feel his presence again. It's not until we embrace being good that we are free from the endless, vicious cycle of perfection.

When we look to Jesus and see that grace, we are able to extend that grace to ourselves. The problem is that most of us women do not look to Jesus, and so we cannot even fathom his grace, let alone give it to ourselves. So what does it look like when we try to change that? There are three verses I always come back to when I find myself obsessing about how my body has changed and is no longer "perfect":

Whatever you do, work at it with all your heart, as working for the Lord, not for human masters, since you know that you will receive an inheritance from the Lord as a reward. It is the Lord Christ you are serving. (Colossians 3:23–24)

So whether you eat or drink or whatever you do, do it all for the glory of God. (1 Corinthians 10:31)

Therefore, my dear brothers and sisters, stand firm. Let

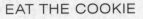

nothing move you. Always give yourselves fully to the work of the Lord, because you know that your labor in the Lord is not in vain. (1 Corinthians 15:58)

We must deny ourselves the worldly Perfection Pursuit to pursue Jesus. Everything we do must be for the glory of God and not for the glory of ourselves or for what the world says we should be glorifying. Loving God with all our mind, heart, and soul will draw us into his presence and allow us to see when we're giving in to the world and need to make a change. In turn, when we draw into his presence and begin to make changes, we are able to get a little tongue-tingling taste of his grace, truly understand it, and be able to pass that grace on to our soul. That is when we have arrived at excellence.

Memorize these verses. Write them down. Stick them to your forehead. Do whatever you need to do to remind yourself of them when you catch yourself opening the gate to the dark and scary path of perfection.

Except maybe don't actually stick them to your forehead. Maybe your bathroom mirror or something.

It's not going to be easy, but it's going to be worth it. The enemy is going to be bugging you full force when you begin to draw closer to the Lord and lay down your worldly pursuits at Jesus's feet. I know the enemy threw some pretty nasty lies at me, telling me I was losing my worth and value. Remember, he knows that fear is at the root of any kind of Perfection Pursuit, so don't be alarmed if some of those ugly fears deep within your soul start coming up and become really, really real. The enemy is crafty and can make you believe that your fears are coming true, but fear is just False Evidence Appearing Real, so you just have to hold on and know that they're big fat lies. Use the verses you just memorized. The more you can fight lies with God's truth, the easier it will be to loosen your grip and let perfection slip through your fingers.

I love how 2 Corinthians 5:17 says, "Therefore, if anyone is in Christ, the new creation has come: The old has gone, the new is here!" When we spend time with Jesus, we are made new. No matter where we are in our life journey, God washes us clean and makes us a whole, new person when we are in him. I never thought I would feel this way, but I can tell you right now that I feel like a new person—a new person with Christ back in her life. We can lay down our desires and pursuit of perfection at the cross, wrap ourselves in God's grace, and allow ourselves to begin to strive for excellence.

If we pursue perfection, we will miss out on what God has for our lives. Perfection is that all-consuming quest that has us look to ourselves for satisfaction. When we look to ourselves for satisfaction in combination with not extending grace to our own soul, we are too busy looking down, not up. Have you ever tried to walk around looking down? You miss out on all the wonderful things around you and probably hurt yourself by walking into a few walls. Walking the Perfection Pursuit is just like that. We miss the amazing things around us because we are so focused on this one—usually insignificant in the grand scheme of life—thing. We also hurt ourselves by not letting ourselves experience the grace that God has for us.

If I had kept listening to the world telling me I needed to continue to change my body and put fitness above all else, I would have missed out on God's best for me. I would have been too busy lifting weights and eating purse chicken to stop and realize that this wasn't what God wanted for me. I would not have made the scary choice to give up the gym, start eating a whole lot more food, and gain weight so that I could truly lay down my body at the foot of the cross, leaving my pursuit of worldly perfection behind me, and walking into the full joy and freedom that I am now experiencing.

What might you be missing in your quest for a big, beautiful, perfectly decorated home? Are you missing time with your kids or your husband, which will give you so much more joy than matching pillows (promise!)? What about your pursuit for a perfect 4.0 GPA? Are you missing some fun outings with your friends that would create more joyful memories in your life? I guarantee you won't look back ten years from now and say, "Remember that time when I got an A in algebra? Ahhh, good times." You'll remember the times spent with your loved ones when you laughed so much your face felt like it was going to fall off your head.

You know what's funny? After we leave that pursuit of perfection behind, it's usually so much clearer to see how imperfect and messy it was. As they say, "Hindsight is 20/20," and it is so true. I look back on that phase of my life, and I can see everywhere I went wrong and how all the things I was chasing were so insignificant. I also understand now why I still felt like I wanted more—because God wasn't a part of the picture. I'm not telling you it's going to magically get easier. Pursuing excellence is still going to be messy and imperfect too because, girlfriend, that's just life. I always tell people, "If it isn't messy, you're doing it wrong." I mean, that's usually in the context of eating some ribs or something saucy and good, but we can totally apply the same saying to life. The difference is that our new excellent (not perfect!) selves are okay with a little mess and a few (or a lot) of mistakes along the way.

And not only will we be okay with a few little messes and mistakes along the way, we will be satisfied, because as Isaiah 58:11 says, "The LORD will guide you always; he will satisfy your needs in a sun-scorched land and will strengthen your frame. You will be like a well-watered garden, like a spring whose waters never fail." Did you catch that? *He* will satisfy your needs in a sun-scorched land (our culture and the media are pretty sun-scorched if you ask me!) and *strengthen you*. Perfection will never keep you satisfied. You will only be wanting more, more, more when perfection is your end goal.

In this book we will dismantle the Perfection Pursuit and gain tools to come back to our healthiest, whole selves. We will learn to embrace imperfection, pursue excellence, and learn to love and accept the way God made us and the life that he created for us without comparison, guilt, or shame. At the end of each chapter you will find Bible verses to help you on this journey and to help you renew your mind and align your thoughts with Christ. The end of each chapter will close with a recipe and a workout to really integrate your healthy body, mind, and soul.

When we find wholeness in the Lord, *he* will satisfy all your needs, strengthening you to resist the enemy when he tries to lure you onto the dark and creepy path.

Remember, that path leads to cobwebs in your hair.

This path may seem dark and scary and unknown at first. But grab my hand, girlfriend, because we're going to walk right into the arms of Jesus one step at a time.

FOR YOUR TOOLBOX

He satisfies the thirsty
and fills the hungry with good things.

—PSALM 107:9

I will refresh the weary and satisfy the faint.

—JEREMIAH 31:25

Then Jesus declared, "I am the bread of life.
Whoever comes to me will never go hungry, and
whoever believes in me will never be thirsty."

—JOHN 6:35

BREAKFAST RECIPE

PESTO HUMMUS EGG TOAST

Toast is all the rage right now! It's the perfect
canvas to put so many things on and is the ideal
crispy base. This toast blends Middle Eastern and
Italian flavors with hummus, pesto, and cheese,
and it's a taste sensation that is sure to get you
out of bed in the morning! It's very easy, so it's
great for busy mornings, and the combination
of protein, fat, and carbs will keep you full until
lunch!

Ingredients

1 large egg
1 tablespoon traditional hummus
½ tablespoon jarred pesto
1 slice of bread (I usually use whole wheat)
1 teaspoon Parmesan cheese
Sea salt

Directions

1. Bring a medium pot of water to a boil. Once boiling, *gently* place the egg into the pot. Cook according to the pro tips on the next page.
2. While the egg cooks, stir together the hummus and pesto. Additionally, toast your bread.
3. Once the egg is cooked, drain the hot water out of the pot and add cold water to cover the egg. Let the egg sit for 5 minutes to cool.
4. Spread the hummus mixture all over the toast. Peel the egg and slice it with a sharp knife. Spread the slices over the hummus. Finally, sprinkle with the Parmesan cheese and a pinch of salt.
5. Devour!

PREP TIME: 5 minutes
COOK TIME: 10 minutes
SERVES: 1

Pro Tips!

1. I like my eggs just a little below hard boiled—where the yolk has a little bit of softness but is mostly firm, so I cook my eggs for 7 minutes 30 seconds. If you want them runnier, cook less (around 7 minutes), or more firm, cook more (8–9 minutes). You may need to experiment to get your ideal cook time.

2. If you want to be extra, you can butter the toast before spreading on the hummus. Extra yummy!

BODY-BUILDING WORKOUT FOR LOWER BODY

Do you want to gain muscle in your lower body? This workout is for you! Typically, in my own training, I like to have one strength-based workout and one size-based workout for each body part during the week. Fewer reps with heavier weights produce an increase in strength over time, whereas slightly lighter weights with middle-of-the-road reps (like 8–12) produce size. This is how I see the most success and growth over time. We're going to do an in-the-gym workout that is going to help increase the overall muscle size in your lower body. There's also a little bit of abdominal work, since the abs provide stability for much of the lower body work that you do!

A range of 8–12 reps gives you a little bit of wiggle room.

So maybe you hit 12 reps with a weight for one of the exercises for the first set, but only 10 reps with the same weight on the second set; that's okay. As long as you are gradually building strength week to week and are working your muscles almost to failure, you are doing it right.

Working the muscles almost to failure means that the last rep that you do in each set is *hard*, but not impossible to complete. You should not have to drop the weight during the last rep because you can't finish it. But you should not be able to do another one after you've completed the last rep.

For each of these exercises, do 3 sets with 60–90 seconds (as noted next to each movement) of rest between each set before moving on to the next exercise. For example, finish 1 set of 8–12 Bulgarian squats, rest for 90 seconds, do another set of 8–12 reps, rest for 90 seconds, and then do a final set of 8–12. After resting for another 90 seconds, move on to the leg press and continue.

This workout should take you around an hour to finish. Make sure to do some dynamic stretching (active movement) before you begin, to warm up your muscles. I also recommend doing each exercise a couple of times with very light weights to prep your muscles before working with heavy weights. Take care of your body, and it will take care of you!

If you don't know what an exercise looks like, YouTube has tons of amazing videos that will show you form. Form is always first!

The Workout

BULGARIAN SQUATS: 3 sets, 8–12 reps, 90 seconds rest
LEG PRESS: 3 sets, 8–12 reps, 90 seconds rest
BARBELL HIP THRUSTS: 3 sets, 8–12 reps, 60 seconds rest

WALKING LUNGES (WITH DUMBBELLS OR BARBELL): 3 sets, 8–12 reps, 60 seconds rest

CABLE PULL-THROUGHS: 3 sets, 8–12 reps, 60 seconds rest

SEATED CALF PRESS: 3 sets, 8–12 reps, 60 seconds rest

ANY AB EXERCISE YOU LIKE: 3 sets, 8–12 reps, 30 seconds rest

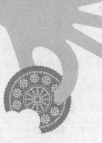

CHAPTER 2

FIND YOUR WORTH

When you learn how much you're
worth, you'll stop giving people
discounts.

—ANONYMOUS

I walked down the stairs, heels on, hair and makeup done, and ready for my date. I went to grab my coat when I heard my dad's voice come out of his office off the entryway, "What's this one's name now, Taylor?" he asked my teenage self. "I can hardly keep up with all your boyfriends these days. There's always a new one. I'm just going to call them all 'Loser Boy' from now on because they never last long anyway."

"Loser Boy." The name for any guy I brought home. When you're on five-plus dating sites at a time and going out with a new guy every week, I guess it makes sense to just group them into one name. I couldn't help myself. The excitement of meeting men on the internet, going on a new date every week, and feeling beautiful and sexy was enticing.

It made me feel needed. It made me feel wanted. It made me feel worthy.

Just like "perfection," I think "worth" is a word that can make us all squirm. We see pretty images all over Instagram alongside sayings about how worthy we are just as we are right now, but when we get off the 'gram and actually live IRL (in real life), what does that actually mean? What is our worth, and where do we find it? Can we will it into existence if we just speak "worth" into the universe? Do we find it in some particular body size? Do we find it in our bank accounts or when we achieve the perfect dream life and family?

Now if I asked you if you were worthy, I'm thinking that your knee-jerk reaction would be to say yes, because very few people would either admit they don't think of themselves as worthy or even know that they don't think of themselves as worthy. I was in the latter camp. I didn't even realize that the way I was living and what I was chasing were directly linked to feeling worthless. Sometimes we cover up these deep, dark, scary feelings about ourselves with that Perfection Pursuit that we talked about because deep down we think that walking down that dark, creepy path will end in a happy fairy-tale forest of self-worth and value and confidence. But girlfriend, let me just be real with you for a sec here: fairy princess forests are not where that path goes.

If you have fallen into the "not knowing you don't know your own worth" camp, then you probably don't even realize that the world has made you feel less than or brought your worth and value into question. I know that I personally don't wake up and say, "Okay, Taylor, how are you feeling today? Do you feel your worth? Do you feel valued?" Feeling our own worth and value often are not things we realize we are missing.

Until we know what it's like to feel it.

Culture and the media tell us that once we have the perfect body, the perfect man, the perfect job, the perfect family, life, kids, or even dog, we will finally have it all. We will feel confident. We will be an "I am woman, hear me roar" kind of lady. Deep down inside our souls we think these things will fulfill us, even if we don't realize it. So we begin to look outside ourselves to find that worth, completely forgetting that the author of worth and perfection is only seen when we look up and not out. We fall into that vicious, never-ending cycle of the Perfection Pursuit only to continue to feel imperfect, unlovable, unvalued, and totally devoid of worth.

In my own journey to self-acceptance and finding my worth in who God says I am, I tried to find my worth in so many different ways. It started with thinking the perfect body would make me feel confident. People would think that I was really awesome and fun and amazing to be around if I was fit.

You read about the purse chicken, the arguments, and the lack of fun nights out. You weren't even my friend at that time, but you already know that I was in no way, shape, or form any fun to be around. It didn't matter how "awesome" my body shape and form were.

You know what's funny? The more weight I lost, the more the number on the scale plummeted, there were more foods I felt "strong" for not eating, and the harder I felt I needed to diet and exercise, the more I actually felt worthless. I didn't feel like a better version of myself, because there was always more weight to lose or more muscle to gain. I didn't feel confident, and I definitely did not have it in me to roar.

Not coincidentally, I also felt further and further away from God, my creator, which also made me feel like I was less worthy. I wasn't achieving the perfect body, and I wasn't close to my savior. I felt like I couldn't do anything right. At times, I even felt like I had to belittle other people who were the "opposite" of me to give myself value. I would poke fun at my family for eating "bad, unhealthy" food so that I would feel better. This went beyond food too.

When I was building my blogging business at the same time as I was really struggling with food, I looked down my nose at people who didn't work twelve hours a day every day of the week. But my own hustle was empty. Really, I just felt like a failure because I was never achieving what I wanted, and I wasn't living a fun, free life. I was miserable, alone, wrapped in fear, and constantly working, and I still wanted more, more, more. This is totally *opposite* of what culture and the media said would happen.

Remember those stick-thin models who influenced my desire to lose weight? They looked *so* happy and *so* confident. Yet, the more I looked like them, the less I felt what they seemed to be exuding. Chasing the perfect body slowly led me to a place of darkness and despair. I wanted this big life, but I felt so small. Around and around the cycle went while I kept hoping that at some point I would arrive and feel whole.

Now, I won't lie to you and say I always felt worthless. The enemy knows what lies to tell us to give us a little high and restore that feeling of confidence and value so we continue chasing perfection. When I turned my hobby blog into a business and felt successful, I definitely felt worthy at first. Which, of course, only lasted so long before I felt totally burned out. When I jumped from man to man, I definitely felt value and worth tied into being desired. But that only lasted so long too. Of course, there were times when my body made me feel worthy as well. I can vividly remember a moment when my trainer at the time put a photo of just my midsection on his Facebook page and everyone commented on how lean I was. In times like those I felt confident and sexy and absolutely worthy.

But that feeling of value lasted about as long as that photo stayed up on his newsfeed, and soon I was back feeling like I could never measure up. The enemy knows this about us. He knows that we will chase something until we find that it is no longer serving us, then we begin to think there has to be *more* than this. More than searching for value and meaning in something outside of ourselves. And this freaks him out. Remember, "Your enemy the devil prowls around like a roaring lion looking for someone to devour" (1 Peter 5:8). He does not want you looking inward, and he definitely does not want you looking up. He wants to keep you as far as he possibly can from God, just like he was doing wo me at this time in my life. So he keeps you stuck, looking to the next thing to find your worth. Whether it's trying some new fitness craze or diet, starting a social media platform and trying to get the most likes, or comparing ourselves to the other mothers at school, he knows how to keep us trapped, and that's where I found myself.

The continual restriction of food, long hours at the gym, and total body obsessiveness never made me feel any more valuable, and so I began serial dating. There were a few years where I could probably have been the spokesperson for internet dating. Not that there is anything wrong with internet dating; it's where I met my husband! At that time, my dating life was not so "Christian," and I knew I wasn't looking for something lasting. I was on every dating site known to man and made sure to bolster my profiles with all my pretty modeling pictures and to talk about how much I liked to lift weights and eat "clean." This definitely wasn't attracting a lifelong mate or a man who could lead me back to Jesus, so I just became a bit of a "man hopper," hopping from "loser boy" to "loser boy."

This felt good to me on the surface. My "hot body" and effort were being seen! Men wanted me. They desired me. I began to associate those feelings and relationships with my own worth, again looking out and not up. I remember a specific time when a boyfriend told me I had a "J.Lo booty," and I felt like I had achieved something totally worthwhile. I defined myself by those comments about my physical appearance, and I had to have a constant waterfall of those compliments raining down on me to feel good about myself.

I kept giving pieces of myself away to these men, thinking somehow that would make me whole. But girlfriend, can we just take a moment to do some math? I know, you didn't sign up for this, but I promise it'll be really simple. If we're being logical here, how does giving away pieces of ourselves—to relationships, beauty, body, grades, wanting to be a supermom, or anything else that we try to find our worth in—equal wholeness? Subtracting from yourself can never equal more.

I didn't realize I was looking to my attractiveness to find my worth until I met my now-husband, Caleb, or Mr. FFF as I affectionately call him on my blog and on the 'gram. He was the man who *truly* loved and valued me above all else, for better or for worse, for richer or poorer, you know the drill. This is also how God loves us and loved me *all* the time, I just was so far away from him that I didn't realize I had this kind of love and affection all while I was looking for it in earthly men.

Although Caleb loves me entirely, I still felt like something was missing. It held me back from recovering for so long because I was so afraid he would no longer love me if I got healthy and gained a few pounds. I still associated his love for me with my body. There were many moments spent on the couch crying to him because of this. The poor man probably wondered what he got into when he said, "I do." I wasn't able to see how freedom would affect our marriage in amazing ways beyond my body, like going on date-nights, or not exercising on vacation, or not berating my husband when he ate a cookie. My brain still associated thinness with worthiness, even though both my husband and God love me for me. I felt like I had to keep striving to find this elusive worth.

Just like the Perfection Pursuit, trying to find your worth in what the world says you need to be just keeps you enslaved to the crazy cycle. You might not have looked to relationships or thinness. I also looked to my job, my bank account, and my number of social media followers. Maybe you look to similar things, or maybe it's your family, education, or something else. Whatever it is, we are all prone to giving people discounts. When we give people discounts, we try to change who we are or force ourselves to do things that don't make us happy because we're afraid of the outcome if we don't. Will people like us? What will people think? It all comes down to searching for worth in the wrong places.

The world thinks being worthy means having qualities other people recognize, that make them think we are totally awesome and accept us. At our very core, we just want to be accepted for who we *truly* are. We want to be usable. But for some reason, we feel like we need to become a *better* version of ourselves to achieve acceptance and have value.

But what would happen if I told you that you are *already* worthy? *Right here. Right now.* It doesn't matter if you weigh one hundred pounds or five hundred pounds, no matter if the other moms at school think you're invincible or if they think you're just barely holding it all together. Regardless of your relationship status, money-in-the-bank status, the size of your house, or size of your pants, *you* are worthy because God made you worthy. You are "fearfully and wonderfully made" (Psalm 139:14). Scripture doesn't say you will be fearfully and wonderfully made when you achieve whatever thing you think you need to feel acceptable and recognized. It says you are fearfully and wonderfully made. *Right here. Right now.* Just as you are.

Now, I'm not telling you to just throw all your goals out the window and sit around binge-watching Netflix and eating bonbons on the couch all day. Although you totally can do that some days, because bonbons are food for the *soul* sometimes. It's still good to have goals and dreams you'd like to achieve. But when those goals and dreams become all-consuming and become tied to your worth, that's the problem. You'll know they're tied to your worth if you start to feel bad about yourself if you don't achieve them. You'll feel like less of a person. You won't extend to yourself the grace we just talked about. You'll get on the Perfection Pursuit and exchange excellence for perfection.

So what is it for you? Take a moment to press pause and figure out what you're trying to achieve that is tied to your worth. Unfortunately, we're not talking about a simple, single knot. A lot of times these things are intertwined with our feelings of worth like strands of Christmas lights you just throw willy-nilly into a box, without taking the time to separate them. Don't lie. You've taken that shortcut, only to realize what a disaster you created when you open that box next Christmas. It may take some time to unravel what is tangled in with your self-worth, but I'm hoping you're at least starting to get the wheels spinning.

You may not feel recognized or acceptable, but lean in a little closer, girlfriend, 'cause I have a secret for you. If we read the stories in Scripture, we find that God *chooses* people who are weak and don't feel equipped. But when they overcome their feelings of inadequacy and worthlessness and take a step of faith to do what God is calling them to do, God is glorified.

First let's look at Mary, the mother of Jesus. She wasn't some fancy-pants princess who had servants carrying her around all day dressed in couture fashion. She was ordinary. She lacked education. She was poor. She was born into a society where women lacked any kind of respect, so her community would definitely overlook a poor, uneducated girl.

But guess what! An *angel* came to Mary. Society didn't pay any attention to her, but God saw her just as she was, and *he* thought she was so important that he sent an angel to her! And you know what that angel said to her? Luke 1:28 says, "The angel went to her and said, 'Greetings, you who are highly favored! The Lord is with you.'" *Highly* favored. Exactly as she was. Uneducated. Poor. Overlooked by the community. But *highly* favored by God—so much so that she became the mother of Jesus. If the Lord was with Mary, valuing her even though the rest of society did not, we can trust he feels the same way about us.

Then there's Esther. She lost her parents at a young age. She was a Jew in a land ruled by a foreign king. But Esther became *queen*. And when the king decided all the Jews should be killed, God chose this orphan to save the Jewish nation. She stepped out and let her faith be greater than her fear and didn't let her feelings of inadequacy stop her. Through Esther, God smashed the plans of the king's advisors and she became a hero, just by being who she was where she was.

Now let's look at Ruth. She lost her husband in the midst of a famine. Remember, this was a time when women were *nothing* without a husband, and women who were alone struggled to provide for themselves. Ruth was so poor and in such a sad place that the only way she could feed herself was to go into fields that had already been harvested and pick up whatever was left behind. God saw Ruth, saw her courage, her faithfulness, and her kindness, and he gave her another husband, Boaz. Even more, when we look at Jesus's ancestry, Ruth and Boaz were part of his DNA.

In the midst of these three women's lives, when they felt alone, afraid, and totally unusable and worthless, God used them for big, great, *amazing* things, just as they were.

These women didn't argue with God. They didn't say, "Nope, sorry. I don't think I'm really capable of that. I don't feel recognized right now, so how on Earth can I do what you're calling me to do?" In our own lives, this is often how we respond to God without even realizing it. Striving for acceptance and value all the time and never accepting who we are right here, right now, is exactly like saying those words to God. It's like telling him he is choosing the wrong person and maybe he should get his head examined because his judgment is off. I don't know about you, but that's not how I want to respond to the creator of the universe. We need to respond the way Mary responded to the angel: "'I am the Lord's servant,' Mary answered. 'May your word to me be fulfilled'" (Luke 1:38).

If reading those stories still doesn't have you feeling fired up just to be who you are, right now, as you're reading these words, let's just take a scuba dive right into Scripture. I want your noggin to *know* your worth and value to God, so we need to look at what he says about us in Scripture.

When I'm feeling unworthy, unacceptable, or unvalued because one of my goals hasn't been achieved (remember, when we feel this way about goals, that means they are entwined with our own feelings of value), I like to ask myself this short, simple, but *powerful* question: "Is God or culture (the enemy) making you feel this way?" Because the true voice of God will never make you feel any of those things.

For example, in my case, "Did God or culture make you feel that you needed a six-pack to be accepted or happy?" But I couldn't find anything in the Bible about six-packs! In your case it might be "Did God or culture make you feel that you needed a 4.0 GPA?" or "Did God or culture tell you that you needed to have the biggest, best house on the block?" Whatever you insert after "Did God or culture . . . ," I can guarantee that when we look to Scripture we're not going to find any verses that are going to support your need for whatever your thing is to be considered worthy.

That is one of the lies of the enemy because, like we talked about, he knows what will get to you and draw you far away from God. He knows what will rot in your soul without you even knowing it. It's kind of like that bag of spinach we all buy on impulse at the store because *greens*! We should be healthy! And then we all just leave it at the back of the crisper drawer to rot because we actually had no intention of doing anything with it. Our insecurities and feelings of inadequacy, if not addressed, will rot our souls, which leads us to search for that worth and value in places outside of ourselves instead of just looking up and realizing we have value and worth in Christ right here and right now.

Asking ourselves the God vs. culture question can help us begin to untangle the root issues of our feelings of inadequacy and unworthiness. Because if we look to Scripture to find the answer and find nothing, we know that it's coming from culture or our very own inner wrong beliefs about who and what we need to be to be accepted.

One of my favorite passages of the Bible is Matthew 6:25–26, which says, "Therefore I tell you, do not worry about your life, what you will eat or drink; or about your body, what you will wear. Is not life more than food, and the body more than clothes? Look at the birds of the air; they do not sow or reap or store away in barns, and yet your heavenly Father feeds them. Are you not much more valuable than they?"

Birds aren't up in the air worrying about if their wing-style is trendy or if Mr. Hot Bird Man finds them attractive or desirable or if the other birds think they're super fly (pun intended). They're just up there doing their own thing, flying around, and being themselves. And guess what? God values them and takes care of them. And if you're made in the image of God (Genesis 1:26), how much more valuable and worthy are *you* to him just as you are? Not trying to strive or change yourself into some crazy idea society has brainwashed you to believe. Reading this verse was a game changer in my walk with God because it was a time when something "clicked." I finally made the connection that my worth was so wrapped up in what others believed about me that I had avoided looking to Scripture to see what God says about me. When I did, I found that he loves and takes care of me no matter what others think or believe about me.

He thinks you are *so* worthy that he died for you. Romans 5:8 says, "But God demonstrates his own love for us in this: While we were still sinners, Christ died for us." He knows we are inclined to search for worth and value in things that are outward and not upward, yet he still loves and values us so much that he sent his one and only Son to die a painful death on the cross to keep anything from separating us from him.

Aside from looking to Scripture and asking myself the God vs. culture question, there was one more little piece of soul-searching I had to do to unravel my worth. I know we've been doing a *lot* of soul-searching here, girlfriend, but can you stick with me for just a little longer? Grab an espresso, and let's belly flop right on into feeling our worth and value just as we should. No pretty swan diving here, folks. Unraveling our worth is messy and a little painful. If you've ever belly flopped before, you know exactly why I'm making this comparison.

When I was working with a counselor to overcome all the lies I've believed about myself for so long, she asked me a really hard question about why I think having a six-pack, or being lean, or having men think I'm a sex kitten would give me worth.

She asked me to dig deep down into the dark and scary cobwebs of my soul to see if I might have misplaced any judgments on people who are the opposite of those things, or people I would think are unworthy. Those subconscious judgments were keeping me in bondage because, in the depths of my soul, I believed them to be true.

For example, I realized that I believed men only wanted one thing, therefore I *had* to be hot and sexy, or I would never be desired by my husband. I realized that I thought people who weren't all about fitness were lazy and lacking motivation or willpower. All these things are completely untrue, of course. They were judgments society had created, or they came about because of my own wrong thought patterns. But because I believed them to be true at the root of my being, I had to dig up those roots and lay a different foundation—one that didn't include allowing those judgments to define who I thought I had to be.

It's uncomfortable for me to admit those things, and it was even more uncomfortable for me to realize I had those beliefs at my core. But breaking through those areas of bondage and realizing they are from the enemy has been one of the most freeing things in my discovery of my own worth and value. It was also one of the things that drew me back to God. I was able to see that those beliefs were lies and that I had to flip the switch. Once that switch was flipped, my thoughts began to align more with the mind of Christ, and when that happens, we naturally draw closer to him. No longer do I feel accepted and recognized based on fitting in some box I have created for myself based on my thoughts about others. I am *allowed* to be free and whole in my own skin. Right now. Just as God made me to be.

I'm not going to lie to you and tell you it'll be a walk in the mall to do this. I'll be the first to tell you that it's gonna get messy and it won't feel good when you sit down and begin to break down whatever judgments and wrong beliefs you have. You might uncover some parts of yourself that you didn't know you had. And, truly, some you won't really like. But these icky parts are the parts that keep us in bondage—the parts that make us feel "not enough" and keep us searching, searching, searching for anything outside of ourselves to give our lives meaning and value.

It isn't until we take our gazes from outward to inward that we can then go from inward to upward.

FOR YOUR TOOLBOX

For you created my inmost being;
you knit me together in my
mother's womb.
I praise you because I am fearfully and
wonderfully made;
your works are wonderful,
I know that full well.
My frame was not hidden from you
when I was made in the secret place,
when I was woven together in the
depths of the earth.
Your eyes saw my unformed body;
all the days ordained for me were
written in your book
before one of them came to be.
—PSALM 139:13–16

Even the very hairs of your head are all num-
bered. So don't be afraid; you are worth more
than many sparrows.

—Matthew 10:30–31

For we are God's handiwork, created in
Christ Jesus to do good works, which God prepared in advance for us to do.

—Ephesians 2:10

For we know, brothers and sisters loved by
God, that he has chosen you.

—1 Thessalonians 1:4

BREAKFAST RECIPE

CARDAMOM MAPLE BUTTERNUT SQUASH PANCAKES

Butternut squash in pancakes? It's a thing!
Butternut squash is cooked and then mashed with
oat flour, sticky-sweet maple syrup, and a double
dose of spiciness from cinnamon and cardamom
to make a hidden-veggie breakfast you are sure
to love! Even picky eaters will not believe they are
eating vegetables for breakfast. Meal-prep them
ahead of time for busy mornings!

Ingredients

$2/3$ cup + 2 tablespoons mashed butternut
squash (see note on following page)

2 large eggs

2 tablespoons maple syrup

2 teaspoons vanilla

$3/4$ cup oat flour (96 grams)[1]

2 teaspoons baking powder

1 teaspoon cinnamon

$1/2$ teaspoon cardamom

$1/4$ teaspoon salt

Directions

1. Heat a griddle to medium-low heat (about 300 degrees) and rub it with coconut oil or spray with cooking spray.
2. In a medium bowl, whisk together the squash, eggs, maple syrup, and vanilla.
3. Add in the oat flour, baking powder, cinnamon, cardamom, and salt, and whisk until well combined.
4. Pour a scant $1/4$ cup of the batter onto the preheated grill. Cook until the bottom is golden and the sides begin to look cooked, about 2 minutes. Flip and repeat on the other side.
5. Top with butter, syrup, or sautéed apples!
6. Devour!

PREP TIME: 5 minutes
COOK TIME: 5 minutes
YIELD: about 9–10 pancakes

NOTES:

To make my squash, I just cut the squash vertically down the center and scrape out the seeds, then place it cut-side down on a parchment paper–lined pan and bake it at 375 degrees until it is soft, which is about 45 minutes to an hour.

Pro Tips!

1. Don't turn your griddle on too far in advance of cooking your pancakes. This will cause it to become too hot, and the outsides of the pancakes will burn before the insides are cooked.
2. Don't have oat flour? You can put some rolled, old-fashioned oatmeal in a high-powered blender and blend for about 1 minute until fine and powdery.

LOWER-BODY STRENGTH WORKOUT

It's important to incorporate exercises that will both strengthen your muscles and make them grow in size for optimal fitness and health. I typically do one strength-based workout and one size-based workout a week: one each for upper body and one each for lower body. I find this to be the easiest way to hit all your body parts, strengthening them and helping the muscles grow.

Typically, I will put this workout on Monday, with a size-building lower-body workout on Thursday or Friday to give my body lots of rest. Personally, I think you should wait at least 48 hours to work the same muscle group to allow it time to heal. Remember, muscles don't grow when we work them out—they grow during the time when we let them rest and recover!

We're using reps of 5–8 for the workout to promote strength. Lower reps with heavier weights increases strength over time, whereas slightly lighter weights with middle-of-the-road reps produce size. This range of reps gives you a little bit of wiggle room. So maybe you hit 8 reps with a weight for one of the exercises for the first set, but only 6 reps with the same weight on the second set; that's okay as long as you are gradually building strength week to week and are working your muscles almost to failure. You can refer to the workout in the previous chapter to learn what "almost to failure" means.

For each of these exercises you are going to do 4 sets with 90–120 seconds of rest between each set (as noted next to each movement) before moving on to the next exercise. For example, you will finish 1 set of 5–8 front squats, rest for 120 seconds, do another set of 5–8 reps, rest for 120 seconds, another set, rest for 120 seconds, then a final set. After resting for another 120 seconds, you will move on to the leg curl and continue in this fashion.

This workout should take you around an hour to an hour and 15 minutes to finish. As always, make sure to do some dynamic stretching (active movement) before you begin, to warm up your muscles. I also recommend doing each exercise a couple of times with very light weights to prep your muscles before working with heavier weights.

The Workout

FRONT SQUATS: 5 sets, 5–8 reps, 120 seconds rest

SPLIT SQUATS (WITH DUMBBELLS OR BARBELL): 5 sets, 5–8 reps each, 90 seconds rest

LYING LEG CURLS: 5 sets, 5–8 reps, 90 seconds rest

WALKING LUNGE (WITH BARBELL ACROSS BACK): 5 sets, 5–8 reps per leg, 90 seconds rest

CALF PRESS IN LEG PRESS MACHINE: 5 sets, 5–8 reps, 90 seconds rest

ANY AB EXERCISE YOU LIKE: 5 sets, 5–8 reps, 60 seconds rest

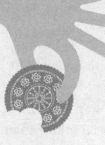

CHAPTER 3

LEARN
TO LET IT GO

I've learned that when you try
to control everything, you enjoy
nothing.

—Anonymous

I opened my door to find yet another package on the doorstep. Another food product to try and share on my Instagram. "This is one of the best parts of my job," I thought. I opened the box to discover this nut butter that looked ridiculously delicious!

I immediately opened the lid and stuck a pinky finger into it. While licking it off my finger, I could hardly contain the huge smile that spread across my face. It was *so* delicious! Scouring the packaging, I looked for the nutritional information. "How much can I have of this today to fit into my calories?" I wondered. It's *so good* that I *need* to make it fit.

To my horror, it was made by a very small company and there was no nutritional information. I put the container into the back of my pantry and told myself I'd just forget about it. There was no point in eating something that would put me out of control of my daily intake, was there?

Sadly, I went back to my fat-free powdered peanut butter—the kind you mix with water and try to tell yourself is just as good as the real thing.

But deep inside we all know it's not.

I like to think I have it all under control. I mean, you already know without even knowing me that I don't. Girlfriend, I'm just gonna let you in on a little secret right now: *no one* has everything under control, and if they do, they're probably not someone you wanna go out for lunch with because they're no fun. I think I've got my business under control, my health under control, my house under control, and even my husband under control. Just kidding on that last one—you can't control those crazy things we call husbands.

And all the women said *amen*.

All of us want to be, or at least appear to be, in control in some way or another; it's a natural desire. Maybe you want to be the head honcho at work and control everything so you end up looking like the star. Maybe you want to be in control of your kids, making sure they're always on their best behavior so the moms think you're a *superstar*. Or maybe, like me, you're one of those "ten-year plan" kinda people who has your whole life planned out because you want to control every aspect. Whatever it is for you, no one wants to feel out of control.

And we're not talking out of control like when your boyfriend broke up with you and you assumed, at the age of twenty, you were doomed to die alone, so you ate an entire box of chocolates in five minutes. Don't look at me like that, I know you did that in your past too. We're talking a *much* deeper loss of control: the kind that draws us away from the One who has everything under control. The kind that makes us feel small. The kind that makes us feel like we're somehow not worthy because we don't have it all together. The kind that fills us with fear of the unknown. We grasp at everything possible so we never have to step into that unknown, and we try to take control of our lives.

Control usually starts with good intentions. It's not a bad thing to want to be great at your job or to have kids who aren't wild and crazy hooligans, or to have plans for your life. Even the Bible tells us self-control is a good thing. Hey, it's one of the fruits of the Spirit: love, joy, peace, patience, kindness, goodness, faithfulness, gentleness, and self-control (Galatians 5:22–23). If it's in the Bible, it has to be a good thing, right?

But you know what is also in the Bible? The enemy. And he is no good.

So why do we try to control? In my opinion, it's for a few reasons. One reason is that humans are prideful! We think we can run our lives the best by ourselves, and we don't want to give God the chance to show us that he can actually do it better. Another reason could be because we're terrified we won't like what God does with our lives if we give him control. We even see Eve trying to take control in the Garden of Eden. She ate the fruit independently of God, and there lies the problem. When we attempt to take control independently of God, things go a little bit crazy.

If you look at the definition of "control" in the dictionary, you might see my face. My husband calls me "Type A+"; I know I am a total control freak. When I started my own business, I couldn't hire anyone to help me, although I was drowning, because that would mean giving up some control. I even had to control the people around me because I thought it might be too risky to be around people and have them find out the real me, the one I thought had no value or worth.

But the biggest area of control for me was food and my body. I controlled my food and exercise, keeping a white-knuckled hold on each bite and each rep so I could control exactly how my body looked. I figured out exactly how many calories to eat, exactly what macros (protein, fat, and carbs), and exactly how many minutes, reps, and sets I had to do at the gym to control my body to be the image of perfection.

Both my mom and my husband used to call me "exercise-mode Taylor" when I was at the gym, because nothing else mattered. If they broke my pace at all, causing me to maybe burn three fewer calories, I would literally have a meltdown on the gym floor. Honestly, when I was in exercise mode, if my husband was working out with me and suddenly passed out, I probably would make sure to finish my sprints before I got off the treadmill to see if he was okay. Hey, it was all in the name of making my life unicorns, rainbows, and cute, fuzzy puppies, right?

Imagine if you walked into your best friend's kitchen and you saw her putting her grapes on a food scale because she wanted to make sure she had the *right* number of grapes, and not too many, because those two extra calories were just *too much* for her body to handle. This was me. I was self-absorbed, no fun to be around, and totally out of touch with who God called me to be. But all I saw was a girl who was totally, 100 percent in control.

Or so I thought.

Let's backtrack a bit for a second. Like, back to when we ate a box of chocolates because we thought our time was up at age twenty. That boyfriend who broke up with me at age twenty was my "trigger." Now, I'm not a shrink, nor am I someone who had a broken childhood that led to my issues. I feel very grateful that this is not the case, and I know if that is your story, God can rewrite your ending and use that mess for your message. Those of us who feel the pressure and weight to control an area of our lives typically have a trigger. It might be something as small as something someone said to you. For example, "My gosh, your kid is just a wild child, isn't he?" But it might be as big as a piece of your life that you thought was secure crashing down. The latter was my trigger.

After I recovered from my eating disorder, it was *full* recovery. No weird weighing of grapes, none of that purse chicken, no figuring out exactly how many minutes on the StairMaster it would take to get the cellulite off my butt forever. This is partially because we all know cellulite isn't going anywhere no matter how much kale we eat, but mostly because the StairMaster is evil, and even one minute on it is *too long*. Life was free, it was full, and it was vibrant, and I felt out of control of it in the best possible way. Then the switch flipped.

I was dating this guy, let's call him Bob because no one names their child Bob anymore, and I thought he was "the one." I had our life planned and everything was just fallin' into place. Until he *broke up with me*. Out of the blue. Totally unexpected.

61

Cue boxes of chocolate, romantic movies, girlfriends texting you about how much of a loser he was anyway, and everything else we did at the young age of twenty when this sort of thing happened to us.

That picture-perfect life that my watched-way-too-many-chick-flick-movies brain had dreamed up was shattered into a million pieces in five minutes. Everything I had planned for my future—from the white picket fence to the fluffy little dogs—had now turned to visions of sitting alone on my couch, watching daytime TV, and playing with my seven cats. I felt scared. I felt alone. I felt like my life was no longer perfect. I assumed I was not worthy of being a girlfriend. I felt angry with God. He knew how badly I wanted to get married. He knew I would be a darn good wife. I could cook! I took care of myself! Parents always liked me! How could he take something away that I so desperately wanted and that would make me happy? I felt like every part of my life was spiraling out of control.

Of course, my current self would have told my twenty-year-old self to put on her big-girl panties because no one is ending up with seven cats and dying alone just because they don't have a man in their life at twenty.

Can you identify with me, though? You're just groovin' along in life, feeling like it's going swell, and then—*wham*—something falls right out of the sky and shakes up everything you thought you knew and leaves you absolutely spinning. That moment is your trigger. That's the moment you want to identify so you can take back control of your life. Actually, it looks more like giving *up* control. But I don't want to scare you away just yet. Grab my hand, girlfriend, and let's keep going.

That shake-up made me start grasping at whatever I could

control to get back that feeling of peace and stability in my life. Because I was angry at God and felt far away from him, it didn't click that going back to him would offer the peace and stability I needed. Since I had an eating disorder in my past, for me that was food and exercise. This is when I found that trainer who would put a picture of just my abs on social media. I'm not going to go into the nitty-gritty here, but we're talking years of weighing grapes and not eating cookies because I was so good at "self-control" that I didn't need those cookies at Christmas.

It's easy for us to justify wanting to be in control because, like I said before, self-control is a fruit of the Spirit. God *wants* us to have self-control. Therefore, we think we are doing the right thing by looking inward to control our lives. If we go back to the "no cookies at Christmas" example, I thought I was a pretty awesome person for being able to control myself around cookies. People commended me for it. They told me they wished that they could be like me. But what they didn't know was that I was thinking about those cookies *all day*, wishing I could just learn to *let go* of control and eat one. I was yelling at God in my mind for making me think of cookies all the time. Why couldn't he just make me not think about food so my life would be so much easier? People didn't know I often said I wouldn't wish what I went through in my brain on anyone. What I didn't realize was that the control I praised myself for was actually controlling *me*.

Typically, at least for me, when I feel like I have it all together and I'm totally in control is usually when I'm the most *out* of control. When we're at our prime at work, killing it and working all the hours, our social and family life can be getting a little out of control. Or maybe you're working so hard on that master's degree you've let your own self-care become nonexistent and out of control. I thought I had my food and exercise and my body *totally* under control, but I didn't realize it was controlling me.

I had obsessive thoughts about food all day long. When would I eat? What would I eat? How many grapes would I be able to have? Would I get hungry and have to ignore it because it wasn't "time to eat"?

I could never go away for a weekend unless the hotel had a gym because I *had to* work out, and missing one workout would turn me into a balloon overnight.

Sitting in that bar bathroom eating purse chicken so that I wouldn't gain one *ounce* overnight.

Those crazy things I held so tightly to make sure my body would be perfect and desirable actually had a hold over *me*. Wanting to achieve that body and doing whatever it took to get there began to control every single thought and every single action. I can tell you from personal experience, being controlled by control itself is probably the least fun and least life-giving thing you could do to yourself, no matter how much you tell yourself that you are doing it to have the best possible life for yourself or be the best possible version of you.

I knew God wanted to have control of my life, but I was still so frustrated with him over the break-up incident that I didn't even want to acknowledge that he was there, trying to get me to give up my life and give it back to him. You might not have gone through a breakup, but I imagine there has been a similar incident in your life when you were angry with God and tried to run the other direction, pretending like you could get everything under control by yourself.

When I say the word "slaves," you probably think of people from the distant past who were run by masters and had no freedom, and you're wondering why I am bringing them up right now. But did you catch that? Slaves are run by masters and have no freedom. Has there been a time in your life when you've been caught in a sin cycle, striving for something that will make you feel like you have worth and value, like I was when I was on that dark and scary Perfection Pursuit? Then you have been a victim of slavery, and control has been your master.

Don't be glum, chum, because that's not where the story ends. Control doesn't have to have mastery over you. Isaiah 61:1 says there will be freedom for the captives and the prisoners will be released from their darkness. That means you! That means me! Jesus came for our freedom. He doesn't want us to be bound by the shackles of control and slaves to the desires the devil places within our hearts.

Can I tell you something? The enemy, that pesky guy who is prowling around like a roaring lion wanting to devour you, is the one who places the need to take control of our lives in our hearts. He knows *God* is in control, but he doesn't want *us* to know that. And so the crazy control cycle continues. Can I tell you something else? Our need for control is rooted in some of the things we've already talked about, like a need for perfection and for a feeling of worth. When you feel like you don't have it all together, do you feel like things are going perfectly? Do you feel super valuable? That's a big, fat *nope*. That drive for perfection and value is what leads us down the dangerous path of control, landing us in the shackles of slavery and unable to see any way out.

That's when we ask, "Did God or culture tell me that I needed to be in control?"

And we realize there is a way out of this control culture. It just looks different from what we expected.

It looks like a man on a cross.

Jesus broke our slavery when he died for us, extending his grace and mercy to cover our sin of trying to take control. Second Corinthians 5:17 says, "Therefore, if anyone is in Christ, the new creation has come: The old has gone, the new is here!" And I love what Paul says in Romans 6:17–18: "But thanks be to God that, though you used to be slaves to sin, you have come to obey from your heart the pattern of teaching that has now claimed your allegiance. You have been set free from sin and have become slaves to righteousness." We no longer need to live in the control cycle, letting it have mastery over us so we continue on the Perfection Pursuit. We are now slaves to righteousness.

And now you're confused. We were just talking about how we want to get *away* from the slavery of control, but now we've just become slaves to something else? Girl, I know it sounds *super* backward, but being a slave to righteousness is the only kind of slavery we want! James 1:25 says, "But whoever looks intently into the perfect law that gives freedom, and continues in it—not forgetting what they have heard, but doing it—they will be blessed in what they do." Being a slave to the will of God allows us to enter into the freedom and fullness of life he wants for us.

When I eventually got over my anger at God, came back to him, and walked through healing, I would read Scripture telling me to not worry about what I would eat. Not worrying about what to eat was a law of God I began to follow, and because of my obedience to that law, I was able to experience freedom and a fullness of life. The same goes for you too. Whenever you walk through life following God's laws, you will find that your life opens up and your freaky, controlling self starts to slowly die.

And while that all sounds well and good, how do we get there? You want to look intently into that perfect law and do it, but how do we actually do that?

Girlfriend, I've got you.

Two other driving factors in an addiction to control, beyond seeking value and perfection, are fear and trust.

Fear is a pretty obvious one. We fear what will happen if we don't control things. I feared what would happen to my body if I didn't control everything I put into my mouth or do every exercise every single day. You might fear what people will think or say if you allow your kids to actually be kids and run around like crazy, wild animals. Or maybe you fear that your life will turn to shambles if you don't have every detail of the next ten years planned out. You get the picture. At the root of every control problem is a fear problem. Fear of being thought "less than." Fear of being found worthless or lacking in value. Fear of not being enough. So we latch onto control. Isaiah 41:10 says, "Do not fear, for I am with you; do not be dismayed, for I am your God. I will strengthen you and help you; I will uphold you with my righteous right hand." This is a verse I repeat to myself every single day (sometimes multiple times a day) because if we allow ourselves to truly believe that what God says is true, we can rest in knowing we should not fear anything because he has us. He will strengthen us. We do not need to control. We just need to know the truth and allow that truth to set us free (John 8:32).

Now, let's talk trust. Don't worry, I'm not going to go all psychobabble on you and try to get down to the root of your trust issues here. But I am going to let you in on a secret. Our control issues also stem from misplaced trust. In my own life, and I'm willing to bet this goes for you too, I have put my trust in my *own* abilities. I felt God had somehow broken trust with me when he took away that relationship, and so I looked at my ability to control my body and my weight and started trying to control things like my job, my marriage, and my living situation. All of it. When we put our trust in ourselves, our status, our wealth, or anything else that is of this world, we are not putting our trust in the God who never fails.

James 4:7 says, "Submit yourselves, then, to God. Resist the devil, and he will flee from you." Did you catch that? If we submit ourselves to God, the devil will *flee from us*. The enemy places the seeds of doubt about God in our heart, making us turn inward, giving in to fear and control. If we submit to God, the enemy has no power. But submitting to God means you have to trust God's plan for your life, family, body, relationships, and everything else.

I'm not going to tell you I'm an ace at this. To be honest, I am pretty bad at trusting God most of the time. I've gotten a *lot* better with trusting him with my body and fitness routine, knowing that whatever happens to my body if I listen to it when it's hungry or too tired to work out is part of the way he designed me. But I'm still pretty awful at trusting him in areas like finances and job security. Giving up control and entering a place of trust is absolutely terrifying, but it's always so incredibly worth it.

Look at the Israelites. Although they were slaves in Egypt, at least they knew what life was going to look like. And so often this is us. We don't love being slaves to control, but it's easier than giving up that control, entering into trust, and walking into the unknown. But you know what? They did it. They left everything they knew to wander around and around in the wilderness for *forty years*. Moses led them on a pretty indirect route, and the Israelites must have been *super* confused, and they doubted Moses. Was he leading them into a trap? Why was everything taking so long? In Exodus 14:11, they eventually even started complaining to Moses that they wanted to go back to Egypt and back to their bondage. Isn't that just like us too? We may allow ourselves to step out in faith and trust God, but as soon as things aren't smooth sailing and aren't going the way we think they should go, we start grabbing back control and falling back into becoming its slave.

God, though, he knows the bigger picture. He knew the Israelites would have to wander and wander, and then, just when they thought they were done wandering, wander some more. He knew Pharaoh would come back after them. He knew they would grumble and complain and want to go back to their regular old bondage. But he *also* knew they would get to the Promised Land.

And they *did* enter the Promised Land. Although they had their moments, they stepped out in faith, trusting God would not lead them astray, and he didn't. They became free people and were no longer slaves.

We may not be actual slaves like the Israelites, but we are slaves to control. If we want to be free, we must truly submit ourselves to God, trusting him in *every* facet of our life. Soon, the devil will flee. Our desire to control will flee. And we will become slaves to righteousness.

If you look back at your life, I'm sure there are many areas where you can see times when you've given up control, trusting God to work it out, and he did. The main thing that comes to mind for me is meeting my husband. I met Caleb in the depths of my obsession with controlling my body and letting it define my worth, and he wasn't having any of that. He made me quit working with the trainer who had brainwashed my mind, and I was *not* into that. But, had I not ended that trainer relationship, I can almost guarantee I would still be in that lifestyle. I'd still be sitting in bar bathrooms, eating purse chicken, and worrying about eating one too many grapes. But here I am, married to the man of my dreams, recovering from years of body-image and worth issues, and feeling freedom, life, and joy. I wouldn't have that life, or my amazing husband, if I hadn't given up my desire for control.

My hospitalization was another time when trusting God to work things out was the only way for me to be free. Being told you could die at any second is scary at any age, but at thirteen? It's terrifying. I hadn't even begun living! I was so afraid, but this is when I started to find my own faith because I *had* to trust God. I literally had nothing else. I was a frail, small teen in a dying body, eating and drinking meal replacement drinks in a hospital doorway so everyone could watch me. I had to do this so the nurses could make sure I wasn't trying to hide food or throw anything away. I had to trust he would keep me alive. He did. And now I'm here writing this book while that amazing husband watches Netflix with my adorable puppy. And I'm truly happy.

When are the times in your own life when God has shown up? Write them down! We can use these times as evidence of God's provision and trust he will show up and take care of us when we are feeling afraid. God isn't a one-trick pony. He doesn't just show up once and never again. If you trust him and *let* him show up and take care of you, he will do it.

If you're still struggling with trust, even after looking back at your own life and seeing where God has shown up, I would encourage you to get quiet and get into the Word. I made what I call a "Jesus corner" in my house. It has a comfy, pretty chair with a cute lamp and a cozy blanket, and it's where I go to spend time with Jesus. I retreat to this corner and practice stillness. I dive deep into his Word and ask him to help me trust him. Getting up each morning and asking God to help me experience him each day is something I still practice.

Are you ready for it? Are you ready to let go and let God? I hope so because, girlfriend, life is so much better on the other side!

Maybe you're still a little fearful of letting go. Or maybe you're not even sure what areas of your life have been defined by control, and that is okay. It's not always easy to figure out, so I have a little exercise for you. Usually we push back when someone challenges or threatens to take away the areas of our lives where we are still holding on to control. For example, when I was healing from my eating and body-image issues, I was okay with starting to eat more. I mean, I was really hungry anyway, so that seemed logical. But when my dietitian told me I should also give up exercise for the time being, my immediate response was, "Uh, well, we'll see. I'll keep it for a bit and see if my body gains health and go from there." When she mentioned it, my muscles tightened and my jaw clenched. Even my body screamed no! I was having a fear response to the thought of not being able to control how my body would gain weight if I ate more food. I wanted to keep exercising so that I could force it to be muscle. I didn't trust that God had made my body smart enough to do what it needed to do to be healthy again.

Maybe you don't have someone actually threatening to take away a part of your life like my dietitian did. But if you look deep inside yourself and ask some hard questions, when do your shoulders tighten up? When do your teeth clench? When do you want to dig your heels in and scream nope! No way! I need that in my life. This is probably the area you're still trying to control, where you're putting your trust in yourself and not in the God who is unfailing, who has it all together, and who has it all under control.

Jeremiah 29:11 is probably one of the most quoted verses in the Bible today, but for good reason. It says, "'For I know the plans I have for you,' declares the LORD, 'plans to prosper you and not to harm you, plans to give you hope and a future.'" When we're so busy being wrapped up in our own control, we can't hear God, and we miss out on the life he has planned for us. He doesn't want to harm us. He *does* have a future planned out for us, and looking inside ourselves or trusting in the wrong thing doesn't help us experience that future. When we place our trust not inward but upward, our hearts and minds and desires will align with God, allowing us to accept his plan for our life, body, marriage, friendships, or anything else you can imagine! Aligning our hearts with God is the first step in beginning to trust him and to give up the control we so desperately think we need. Proverbs 16:9 says, "In their hearts humans plan their course, but the LORD establishes their steps." No matter how much planning, striving, or controlling we do, God's will for every area of our lives will prevail. The sooner we trust in that plan, the sooner our hearts will align with God and we will walk in the freedom we desperately need.

I know this is easier said than done. Trusting that God has our life all planned out and that we will actually be okay with his plan is no easy feat. Full surrender is probably the hardest and most scary thing God calls us to. It's easy for us to give up the parts of our lives he calls us to give up that we don't like. But as soon as he calls us to give up the parts of our lives that we do like, that is when we push back. That is when we start to question his plan for us and want to take back the control. Girlfriend, you and I need to try to get back to a childlike faith. You've probably heard this idea many times before, and I do believe it can get misinterpreted to mean blind faith. My definition of a childlike faith is one that is present and in the moment. Kids don't walk around trying to control everything, they just trust that adults will help them and meet their needs. Having a childlike faith doesn't mean we don't have any faith questions, it means we trust God to help us and meet our needs, and that his plan for our lives leads to total freedom. When I was my most controlling self, I was far from in the moment. I was never present, always trying to figure out how I could tweak the outcome of whatever situation I was in to suit my needs. But as I walked through healing, I had to learn to look to God in those moments and draw near to him. I had to have an in-the-moment faith, praying to God during the scary and hard times, asking him to give me a peace I could trust because he had already orchestrated the outcome. Because of that childlike, present faith, I was able to draw close to God and walk into freedom.

I'm not telling you that you should have no goals. Goals are a great thing to have. I still have fitness goals, goals for my business, and goals for my marriage. The difference between control and goals is that control forces you to achieve those goals and elicits a feeling of fear or unworthiness if they are not met. It's all-encompassing, and you define your life by it. The secret is to find balance and to hold our goals with an open hand. This gives us the freedom and peace to be okay if they are not met. To know an unmet goal doesn't change our worth or value. And it allows us to be able to hear the call of God and step into the full, big, and beautiful life he has in store, trusting that he has it all working out for our good (Romans 8:28).

So, girlfriend, let go and let God. No matter what you are trying to control, I can promise you his way is better. No matter how scary and out of control it may feel to give up control, giving your trust to God will have you walking into freedom.

FOR YOUR TOOLBOX

The LORD Almighty has sworn,

"Surely, as I have planned, so it will be,
and as I have purposed, so it will
happen."
—ISAIAH 14:24

In his hand is the life of every creature
and the breath of all mankind.
—JOB 12:10

The LORD does whatever pleases him,
in the heavens and on the earth,
in the seas and all their depths.
—PSALM 135:6

Many are the plans in a person's heart,
but it is the LORD's purpose that prevails.
—PROVERBS 19:21

PRE-WORKOUT RECIPE

CHOCOLATE, ALMOND, AND COCONUT PRE-WORKOUT PROTEIN SMOOTHIE

Getting proper nutrition before your workout is important to give you the fuel to run faster, lift heavier, and just have an all-around better workout! This protein smoothie will take you less than 5 minutes to prepare, so it's great for a quick meal before the gym. It's loaded with healthy fats and protein, with just a little bit of carbs from the honey.

You want to teach your body to burn fat when you work out, so giving it more fat and protein (to rebuild your muscles) in the pre-workout meal will teach it to utilize fat when there isn't an abundance of carbs waiting to be used. The honey adds a little bit of quick-digesting carbs to give your body that little extra energy to burn as well.

This smoothie tastes like drinking an Almond Joy milkshake!

Ingredients

1 cup canned light coconut milk
1 cup crushed ice
¼ cup chocolate protein powder
¼ cup avocado, mashed
2 tablespoons natural creamy almond butter
1 tablespoon honey
1 tablespoon cocoa powder

Directions

1. Put all the ingredients in a high-powered blender and blend until smooth and creamy.
2. Slurp up!

PREP TIME: 5 minutes
COOK TIME: 0 minutes
YIELD: 1 big smoothie

Pro Tips!

1. You can use any protein you want here—whey, plant, egg white—whatever works best with your dietary needs.
2. This makes a big smoothie, so you want to give yourself enough time to digest it before exercising. If you will be exercising relatively

soon after drinking this, you may want to make half the recipe. You don't want to get cramps!

3. If you want to make this a lower-carb smoothie, you can omit the honey and use 1–2 tablespoons of monk fruit, to taste.

UPPER-BODY BUILDING WORKOUT

It's important to balance out the muscles in your upper and lower body by working them equally throughout the week. I typically hit my upper body twice a week and my lower body twice a week—one strength and one building day each. This allows you to increase both your strength and overall muscle size over time.

I've explained the use of different rep ranges to cater your workout to either strength, size, or endurance. Because we're doing another size workout, we're going to be working with rep ranges of 8–12 for each exercise. Just like the lower-body building workout, you have some wiggle room within each set, so you may hit 12 for one set but only be able to hit 8 the next set. This is okay. Just make sure you adjust weights accordingly—going up or down in pounds—to stay within this rep range, going almost to failure. I explained "almost to failure" in the first workout, so you can refer to it for a definition of what this means.

For each of these exercises you are going to do 3 sets with 60–90 seconds (as noted next to each movement) of rest between each set, before moving on to the next exercise. For example, you would finish 1 set of 8–12 standing military presses, rest for 90 seconds, do another set of 8–12 reps, rest for 90 seconds, and then do a final set of 8–12. After resting for another 90 seconds, you will move on to doing standing lateral raises and continue in this fashion.

This workout should take you around 45 minutes to an hour to finish. As always, make sure to do some dynamic stretching (active movement) before you begin, to warm up your muscles. I also recommend doing each exercise a couple of times with very light weights to prep your muscles before working with heavy weights. You never want to jump right into heavy weights, or you risk injury!

The Workout

STANDING MILITARY PRESS: 3 sets, 8–12 reps, 90 seconds rest

STANDING LATERAL RAISE: 3 sets, 8–12 reps, 60 seconds rest

BENT-OVER BARBELL ROWS: 3 sets, 8–12 reps, 90 seconds rest

SEATED LATERAL PULLDOWN (MEDIUM GRIP): 3 sets, 8–12 reps, 60 seconds rest

STANDING DUMBBELL CURL: 3 sets, 8–12 reps, 60 seconds rest

CABLE TRICEP PUSHDOWN: 3 sets, 8–12 reps, 60 seconds rest

CHAPTER 4

SAY SAYONARA
TO FEAR

Fear is a liar.

—Zach Williams

As we drove up to the restaurant to meet some friends for dinner, a lump rose up in my throat. I started to feel panicky. Anxious. Even shaky. Nothing was truly wrong—we were just going on a double date—but everything *felt* wrong.

"I'm going to have to order something scary from the menu so they don't think I look weird," I thought. "I can't get my usual greens, hold the cheese, hold the nuts, and dressing-which-I-won't-even-use-anyway on the side please." Anxiety rising higher. My heart started to thump in my chest.

Deep inside my soul I knew going out for dinner should not elicit such a deep fear to bubble over into my life. "Normal" people weren't so afraid of food, for crying out loud. I could fear things like spiders or clowns, but dinner?

Something had to change.

I like to think I am a pretty fearless person. Travel around the world without a specific plan? Let's do it! Try some strange, foreign food without knowing what it really is? I am in. Unfortunately, those kinds of crazy, exciting, fear-facing events don't happen regularly in real life. I like to think that I am fearless in my day-to-day life: fearless at loving my husband well, fearless at taking risks in my business, and fearless in my faith.

But the truth is, for a very long time, I was not really as fearless as I thought.

In fact, whether I realized it or not, fear was actually the number-one thing separating me from the big, beautiful life God had planned for me. But because of my *I-am-oh-so-fearless* perspective, I truly thought I was, well, fearless. I didn't recognize that perhaps some of the struggles and strongholds in my life could be based out of fear.

Think you're fearless too? Girlfriend, grab a cup of coffee (or tea, or matcha—if you're trendy—or wine, if it's happy hour) because we're about to do some digging. Even if you think you're pretty aware of your fears, everyone can benefit from a little soul-searching. We're going to come out on the other side together. I pinky promise.

Over a decade ago, when I was in the depths of an eating disorder, I was certainly living a fear-based life. I even kept lists of "good foods" and "fear foods." I was so afraid of gaining any weight that I once cried real tears because my dad made me eat one extra blueberry, and another time when he made me eat *one* Rice Krispie. Not a Rice Krispies Treat, mind you. Just one tiny little grain of crispy cereal. If that is not the definition of fear, I don't know what is.

Fast-forward seven years later, and those secret ninja fears (as I call them) had really gotten their icky-sticky little selves stuck in my heart, and I didn't even realize it. It all began with that completely impossible quest for perfection.

You're about to laugh at me, and I am actually laughing at myself right now, because what I am about to tell you is a real-life, what-was-I-thinking moment. I was going on a first date with a guy I really liked. He wanted to go to a restaurant I knew didn't have anything from my "good foods" list. I was terrified, but of course I didn't actually use that word because I was Xena, Warrior Princess and had no fears.

I was also a fitness-queen-ultra-dedicated-perfectionist person, and there isn't anything wrong with having a foods-I-don't-eat list. So you know what I did? I packed some scrambled egg whites in a tiny Tupperware container in my purse, figuring I would order some minestrone soup for my meal and just pretend to eat it. Then I could slip away to the bathroom halfway through dinner and eat the egg whites.

You know what they say about best-laid plans, right? Well, on the drive to the restaurant, my Tupperware lid popped open, and suddenly the whole car was filled with the smell of cooked eggs.

"Did you just *fart*?" my date asked as he quickly rolled down the windows.

I was humiliated. The rest of the drive—and the rest of the date, for that matter—was spent in almost total silence, and there was no second date. Not that I'm mad about that, because he wasn't my amazing now-husband (obviously). But can you even believe that the fear of eating something that could make me gain weight was so real to me that I would do such a crazy thing? Then again, I've already told you about purse chicken, so you probably believe I would do something like that.

But in spite of how embarrassing these stories are, I'm thinking you can probably identify with me. Maybe not with the egg white story, because I am pretty sure I am the only person on Earth that would happen to, but you can identify with doing something totally ridiculous out of dedication to your cause. I always believed that anything justified having a perfect body. After all, if I had the perfect body, everyone would think I also had a perfect life, and maybe you feel the same. Maybe your "ridiculous thing" was choosing work over that relationship. Or maybe it was not being totally honest on a test to ensure you got the perfect grade. Maybe something totally different. But it was all to achieve some kind of façade of perfection.

It's time for some straight talk: Perfectionism, at its very core, is fear. However, our society also praises those who seem to do things perfectly and have everything together. So it's easy to justify your pursuit of perfection. You want to feel like a rock star when your head hits the pillow at night, knowing you did it *all* perfectly.

But what would happen if—*gasp*—you were a *normal* person, a person who made a mistake and was actually not *perfect*? Would people still want to be your friend? My desire for perfection in every area of my life—food, body, work, relationships—was based on the fear that if I wasn't perfect, I would be less valuable in the eyes of the world. And this fear became the controlling factor in my life, the root of all my problems.

First Peter 5:8 outlines exactly how the enemy wiggles his nasty little self into our souls if we are not careful: "Be alert and of sober mind. Your enemy the devil prowls around like a roaring lion looking for someone to devour."

Did you catch that? The enemy wants to devour our very souls—not just snack on them, but *devour*. He wants us to be incapable of living in a way that is aligned with God's truth, the truth that would ultimately lead us to our best, happiest, and most vibrant selves! Truth be told, he did a *really* good job with this in my life. I could not understand God's truth while I was on the Perfection Pursuit because I had believed the lies of the enemy, which made me feel incredibly far from God and did not allow me to live out the life I know he wanted me to live. While I believe a lot of our wrong thinking is from the enemy, I also believe he plants "fear seeds" in our hearts without us even realizing they're there. And those seeds affect us deeply.

As we talked about before, when Moses was leading the Israelites out of Egypt, they actually started to grumble and complain about wanting to go back to Egypt, the very place where they were under bondage and oppression. They were fearful of their future and wandering in the wilderness, so it seemed like going back to the known would be easier than walking into the unknown. How many times do we do this in our own lives? After I recovered from my eating disorder, I was strong, healthy, and 100 percent better for a good seven or eight years. I chose to exercise and move my body because I loved doing it. I ate mostly healthy food, but I did not even think twice about sharing a whole Dairy Queen ice cream cake with two of my girlfriends. (True story. It really happened. Still feel sick thinking about it.) I was happy and whole, truly tapping into the beautiful life God had for me.

But then something switched. The enemy got his sticky little fingers in my brain and started to once again plant those little fears: I no longer felt like I was enough, and I started to give others' opinions and thoughts of me too much value. Before I knew it, I found myself right back there in bondage: tracking calories, fixating on foods, and constantly worried about my weight. I was back in bondage in Egypt.

For you, it might look like going back to an old relationship you know isn't good for you because it feels familiar. Or maybe it's even going back to an old career that doesn't inspire you and light you up, but it makes you feel worthy because you have more power in the workplace. It might even be feeling the desire to have another child when you know it would put a challenge on your marital relationship because having a little person to depend on you makes you feel needed. At some time in our lives, we all have a desire to go back to an old part of life that was familiar and felt safe, even if we know it wasn't the best or healthiest place for us.

In this "Israelite mentality," I convinced myself that my struggles were manageable. After many years of trying to control every aspect of my life, this setback seemed minor. I was able to go out for dinner with Caleb and maybe even have a cocktail or two. I went away for fun weekend trips. I even ate some of my "scary foods." But although it looked like I was making good progress and breaking some of my fears, I knew in my heart it was all a lie.

That meal out with cocktails? I starved myself all day to "save up" calories for the evening.

That weekend away? I killed myself at the gym, some days even doubling up workouts during the week, to make sure I didn't miss a workout while I was traveling.

Those scary foods? They took the place of another meal so they actually didn't "count" as much.

Have you been there? Trying to make changes but still trying to control every aspect of those changes out of fear that maybe you'll change a little *too* fast and not like the outcome? The fear of truly living my life and having my body change still ruled my heart. Deep down, I worried so much about what people would think if I changed that I grasped at any semblance of control I could find to make myself feel comfortable and less terrified that I wouldn't be able to measure up.

And if I am being honest, I still battle with these thoughts today. When I choose to do something I consider to be freeing, I sometimes feel like I am letting myself down. You see that, though? Letting *myself* down. Why do we hold ourselves to such high standards, placing so many rules on our lives that we become fearful of living out exactly who we were meant to be? Why did I tell myself I had to be "fitness-queen Taylor" or "best-blogger-ever Taylor" or "best-wife-of-the-year Taylor?" Why can't I just be Taylor without any kind of fancy-schmancy title attached to it? And why can't you just be, well, you?

Maybe you totally identify with a pursuit of the perfect body, or maybe you've put so much pressure on yourself in your career, relationships, education, or motherhood that your identity is now wrapped up in fear of not living up to your own standards.

It's time to realize that these are *not* our own standards. They're the standards of the enemy. He will wiggle his way into your life, telling you that everything you're doing is for yourself to make your life better. But until we dig deeper and separate his voice from our own voice *and* from God's truth, we're always going to be under the bondage of fear.

When I was really struggling between wanting to be free but also wanting to stay in my comfort zone, someone asked me a very thought-provoking question: "Aren't you currently eating and exercising out of fear, but also not choosing to really live your life out of fear?" What they meant was that the way I was eating and controlling my calories was out of fear of gaining weight. But I was also choosing to not really live my life because of fear of the unknown. Fear that living my life and risking weight gain wouldn't be "worth it." What if the true Taylor wasn't really worth breaking down the walls of fear and anxiety that I'd built around my life?

Looking back now, I know it didn't really make sense to choose the fear in the form of the micromanaging and body obsession that was bringing me no life or joy whatsoever. But at this point in my life, I was so in tune with the enemy's lies about me, and so not in tune with God's truths, that I had somehow convinced myself that choosing that way of living made sense. I wasn't spending enough time—or, really, any time—with God daily, so I wasn't even letting him in to show me the mistake I was making. In reality, my only other choice was also surrounded by fear.

It wasn't until I recognized that although it comes with fear, choosing to walk into God's plan for my life, trusting he has me every step of the way, was the only path possible if I wanted to live a bigger and brighter life.

So if we're going to be afraid anyway, why not choose the fear that has the most potential to lead to life? Choosing any fear is not easy. Trust me, I get it. I've been there, choosing between two fears. But I can promise you that when you step out and chose the fear that leads to life, eventually, once you get through the hard stuff, you will be so incredibly glad you trusted God and took that step from fear into freedom.

In Exodus 14:15, God asked Moses, "Why are you crying out to me? Tell the Israelites to move on." In the same way, God just wants us to *move on* out of fear into freedom. Yep. That's it. Put one foot in front of the other and just start walking, right here, right now.

Are you laughing? Because I'm laughing. Sometimes when I read the Bible, I find myself saying, "Okay, God. Easy for you to say because you're, well, *God*."

You and I both know that when we're living a life that's wrapped up in fear, it's not as easy as simply moving on. When you've lived your life out of fear and made so many choices based on what felt less scary to you in the moment, it's not so easy to just start walking. But there are some things that can help us get started.

First, we have to assess what's false, and there are two ways to do this.

1. CONDUCT A LIFE CHECK

Before we even take one step into Scripture to see what God says about fear and truth, we need to get super basic by conducting a "life check." Life checks can be used whenever you have to make some kind of decision or choice—in my case, often when I'm in a situation where I find myself struggling with food or exercise. You can do a life check in any situation where you're tempted to control your surroundings. Life checks allow you to separate yourself from the situation for just a moment and ask yourself these questions:

1. Am I trying to control this situation to have some sort of perfect outcome?
2. Is controlling this situation giving me life or hindering me from living? In other words, will making this choice help me just survive, or will it help me thrive?

If your answer to the first question is yes, you can bet your bottom dollar that you're currently operating in a place of fear. Fear doesn't always manifest itself in obvious ways, so identifying these moments of fear will be a little tricky at first. You're most likely not going to get a case of the shakes and actually think, *This situation is so scary.* It's going to require a little digging to determine the reasons you are trying to manipulate the situation. When I'm looking at a menu in a restaurant, mentally breaking down each option based on which has the least amount of calories, I have to pause and ask myself, "Why am I trying to figure this all out instead of letting myself instinctively choose what option sounds the yummiest?"

You have to be a "situation sleuth" by learning to identify those situations that are keeping you in bondage and then start working backward to understand the root of that fear. It won't be easy at first, but with practice it will get easier. I promise.

The second question is a bit easier to answer because you just did a super fab job at identifying your fear. Is the situation you fear leading you to a full, happy life, or is it doing the very opposite? Let's go back to the restaurant example for a second. When I'm out for dinner with Caleb and my brain is busy breaking down the calories of everything on the menu, I am usually not listening to a word he is saying to me. Good wife? Nope. I'm more concerned with myself and my own desires than being present and in the moment with my husband. And then after I've ordered some boring salad, nix the cheese, and dressing-on-the-side-thank-you-very-much, I end up looking longingly at Caleb's food the whole time, wishing I was eating that. So I'm still not being present and I'm feeling sad about my choice, which leads to not living this fun date-night to the fullest.

If that example doesn't get you, let me tell you about my honeymoon. A honeymoon should be the best week of your life, right? Sadly, for us, it wasn't. We were at an all-inclusive resort in Mexico and I didn't want to eat any of the desserts or try any of the frosty drinks because—*gasp*—*sugar*! I spent the whole trip wishing I could enjoy all the great options at the resort but instead chose to hunker down in my castle of fear. Add to that, Caleb and I fought every day because he wanted to enjoy all these cool new foods and tropical cocktails with his new wife, but she was just too busy burning calories in the gym or eating another boring salad.

Yep. True story. Basically, I was the walking definition of "surviving, not thriving."

I bet you've been in this situation over and over and over, and you always make the same choice because you tell yourself it's the "right" choice, that maybe it will make you happy this time, or even that it's what you want.

I have a third question for you: When you've made that choice in the past, have you ever gotten the outcome you were hoping for? Has your decision made you feel alive and happy and whole? If I'm trying to decide between a plate of lettuce and a fabulous meal, hoping to attain some level of perfection and worth through that decision, that is a lot of baggage to put on the poor salad. For proof, I only need to look at my past dinner dates. Did I make the healthy choice then? Probably. Did that healthy choice make me feel amazing? Did I enjoy the rest of the date and feel alive and happy and love my husband best?

Sorry to break it to you, but that's a BIG. FAT. NOPE.

If you've been down this road a time or two, and it always leads to the same place—right back to you trying to control the situation out of fear—I can guarantee it's because you are operating out of fear: False Evidence Appearing Real.

How can doing something the same way every time lead to a different outcome *this time*? Girlfriend, I am gonna be straight with you: it's just not possible.

If this fear has never led you to a fuller life in the past, it's time to acknowledge that even though the evidence appears real in the moment, it's likely false.

Another "life check" question would be, "Am I doing something out of fear of what others may think?" Personally, I lived under my own crazy standards, but I also lived under these made-up standards that I *thought* every other person in the world had for me. I didn't realize other people didn't care if I was or wasn't "fitness-queen Taylor" or "best-blogger Taylor." My husband didn't even want me to be the world's most perfect wife all the time. Really, people probably didn't even think much about me at all—unless they were family or friends, of course. Yet the opinions and values of these "other" people who had no real connection to me made such a strong impact in my life. Sound familiar? I can tell you without a doubt that other people don't care if you are the hardest-working person at work, went to the best university in the world, or have kids who behave like angels all the time. If they're close to you, they just care about you being you. And if they're not close to you, they're thinking about you way less than you imagine.

One thing I realized through this, however, is that the fear of others judging us is really *us* judging *them*. At first this probably makes no sense, but hear me out. When we fear others' judgments of us, we are really saying to them, "You don't have the grace of God to love me for who I truly am." We are judging them for having a lack of grace and acceptance, which is usually not the case at all. It's just something we have made up in our minds because we are giving in to the lies the enemy places in our brains—the False Evidence Appearing Real. The enemy doesn't have one iota of grace in his body, so when we look at others through the lens of the enemy's thoughts, it becomes impossible to imagine they would have any grace for our "flaws." So we judge what they don't, and we try to strive for some made-up standard we think they have for us.

We were not designed to live sad, dark existences, being crushed by the pressure of our own standards or the made-up standards we think others have for us. If something is stealing your peace and joy, it's not ever going to bring you the full life Jesus promises in John 10:10. Which leads me to the next tool.

2. FALSE EVIDENCE APPEARING REAL: LOOK TO GOD'S TRUTH

Conducting these life checks and "soul sleuthing" is a really great start. At the very least, life checks help you to start identifying fears in your life that you may not have even known were there. But once you do this, it's time to do a belly flop right into what Scripture says about fear. No tiptoeing over to the side of the pool and practicing your graceful swan dives. We don't have time for that—our life is waiting! We need to get raw and real and begin uncovering what God has to say about fear in our lives because as John 8:32 says, "Then you will know the truth, and the truth will set you free."

If freedom is supposed to be our outcome, which *it is*, then we need to actually *know* the truth we have access to throughout the Bible. In our battle to identify what is False Evidence Appearing Real, the best place to start is by identifying what is truly real (God's words). Once we recognize truth, we'll be so much better equipped to recognize our fear.

Fear seems like the villain, right? But what if fear actually had a purpose? What if fear could be a powerful prompt to push us toward deeper dependence on God? We don't have all the tools we need to break down the walls of the fear fortresses we've built. We need God to come alongside us to hand us the required tools at every step of the journey. And the truth is that sometimes breaking down our self-made walls is a very slow and gradual process. Stone by stone, fear by fear, eventually we will see those walls come down.

I'm not asking you to be a fearless warrior by the time you've finished this chapter. I've been working through my own fears, trying to learn to place my trust in God to hand me the tools to break them down for a long time now. Some days are easy and God and I feel tight in our trust. Some days we don't. Some of your walls may come down quickly, but others may take years. The key is to remember that nothing is insurmountable when it comes to the cross.

Ephesians 2:10 says, "For we are God's handiwork, created in Christ Jesus to do good works, which God prepared in advance for us to do." You see that? It doesn't say, "For we are God's handiwork, created in Christ Jesus to live in the shackles of fear." It says we were created to do God's *good works*, which he has already prepared for us to do. We just have to take a page out of God's playbook with the Israelites and *move on*, trusting that he is going to give us the power and tools to walk from fear to freedom as we put one foot in front of the other. Even if it's half a step. Even if you just kind of shuffle one foot forward. Even if it's the babiest of baby steps. You're taking a step and slowly walking into something more beautiful.

In Exodus 14:13–14 Moses tells the Israelites, "Do not be afraid. Stand firm and you will see deliverance the LORD will bring you today. . . . The LORD will fight for you."

And Joshua 1:9 says something similar: "Have I not commanded you? Be strong and courageous. Do not be afraid; do not be discouraged, for the LORD your God will be with you wherever you go."

Girlfriend, when you've addressed the underlying fears in your life, wondering where on Earth you go from here, Scripture tells you: *You* don't have to go anywhere on your own. God will be with you as you walk head-on into that scary place (even with the babiest of baby steps or a shuffling situation), and he is *fighting* for you. It took me a very long time to realize God was fighting for me and I didn't have to do everything on my own, which is one of the reasons I feel it took me so long to recover. The enemy had me so far away from God, believing I was totally alone, and when you feel alone, the last thing you really want to do is step out into fear.

Psalm 34:4 says, "I sought the LORD, and he answered me;

he delivered me from all my fears." It doesn't say, "I sought the LORD and he answered me once I had the strength on my own for him to deliver me."

To be honest, though, there were times in my life when I would have read that verse in that way. I believed I would only be delivered from my fears when I was strong enough, which was never happening because I was too afraid of my own fear to *be* strong enough. How silly is that? Knowing we don't have to fight the fear that shackles our lives gives us the ability to take that baby step, trusting that God promises us deliverance.

When the Israelites listened to God and moved on, things didn't immediately turn around. Instead of stepping into freedom, they found themselves between the raging Red Sea in front of them and the Egyptian army behind. Talk about an edge-of-your-seat movie moment! There seemed to be no way out. But in spite of their fears, they chose to put one foot forward in faith. God parted the Red Sea, building a fortress of water around them as protection. He then caused the waves to come crashing down on the Egyptians. Just as he delivered them, God will deliver us, even when we're facing a seemingly insurmountable body of water. We have to obey his command to move on in faith and walk through our own Red Sea, trusting that God will cause it to crash down over all our fears.

Psalm 119:86 says, "All your commands are trustworthy." If God is commanding us to not be afraid (Joshua 1:9), and all those commands are true and trustworthy, then we have no choice but to say, "Fear, you are a liar."

FOR YOUR TOOLBOX

Do not fear, for I am with you;
> do not be dismayed, for I am your God.
I will strengthen you and help you;
> I will uphold you with my righteous
> right hand.
> > —ISAIAH 41:10

Peace I leave with you; my peace I give you.
I do not give to you as the world gives. Do not
let your hearts be troubled and do not be afraid.
> —JOHN 14:27

The LORD is my light and my salvation—
> whom shall I fear?
The LORD is the stronghold of my life—
> of whom shall I be afraid?
> > —PSALM 27:1

Be strong and courageous. Do not be afraid
or terrified because of them, for the LORD your
God goes with you; he will never leave you nor
forsake you.
> —DEUTERONOMY 31:6

The LORD is with me; I will not be afraid.
> What can mere mortals do to me?
> > —PSALM 118:6

POST-WORKOUT BANANA CINNAMON PROTEIN RICE PUDDING

After you work out, your muscles need to be refueled! The best way to fuel muscles is by giving them a combination of protein and carbohydrates that digest quickly so they can be shuttled to the muscles faster.

White rice and fruit are both sources of these quick-digesting carbohydrates, and protein powder is a quick-digesting protein, which makes this rice pudding the perfect post-workout meal! Plus, it's easy to make ahead so you can come home and get your fuel on! Don't be scared of the egg white in here; it makes it so creamy and fluffy!

Ingredients

1/2 cup cooked white rice, lightly packed

1/2 cup unsweetened almond milk

1/4 teaspoon vanilla extract

Pinch of salt

1/4 cup banana, mashed (about 1/2 a large banana) + additional for serving

1 large egg white

1/2 teaspoon cinnamon + additional for serving

2 tablespoons vanilla protein powder

Directions

1. In a medium pot, combine the rice, almond milk, vanilla, and salt. Bring to a boil over high heat.
2. Once boiling, reduce the heat to medium and simmer until it just begins to thicken, about 2–3 minutes.
3. Stir in the banana, egg white, and cinnamon, and cook, stirring constantly, until the egg white is no longer visible, about 1 minute.
4. Add in the protein powder and cook until thickened to your liking. I like it cooked another 2–3 minutes.
5. Sprinkle with additional cinnamon and top with additional sliced bananas, if desired.
6. Devour!

PREP TIME: 5 minutes

COOK TIME: 15 minutes

SERVES: 1

NOTES:

To cook the rice, I brought 1½ cups of water to a boil. Once boiling, I stirred in ¾ cup of rice. Then I turned the heat to low, covered the pot, and cooked it for 20 minutes.

Pro Tips!

1. Make a big batch at once so you have a quick and easy post-workout meal for the week!
2. Get creative! Try making this with different spices and different fruits.
3. Depending on how sweet you like your food, you may need to add some honey or maple syrup after cooking.

UPPER-BODY STRENGTH WORKOUT

I've given you an upper-body workout to promote size, but now we want to work on strength! Big muscles look great, but they don't really add much to our lives because they are not truly strong. Doing a program for strength and a program for size will help create this much-needed muscle balance.

It's important to give your muscles at least a 48-hour rest before working them out again. For example, if you're doing the upper-body building workout on Tuesday, you wouldn't want to do this upper-body strength workout until at least Thursday. My typical week looks like: lower-body strength Monday, upper-body strength Tuesday, rest day Wednesday, lower-body size on Thursday, and then the Tabata cardio workout on Friday, with an upper-body size on Saturday. This allows my muscles to rest and recover, and it feels like a really good balance between exercise and rest for my mental and physical state.

I've talked about the different rep ranges and how to tailor them to suit your needs for strength, size, or endurance. Today, we're working with reps of 5–8 to promote strength in our muscles. As always, the reps give you a bit of wiggle room, so you just want to make sure you are staying within the 5–8 rep range for all your exercises. Even if that means you need to decrease your weight for the second, third, and/or fourth sets of the exercise. Remember, muscles do not understand how much you are lifting, only our egos understand that! They understand time under tension and respond well to that, no matter how much the number on the weight says.

For most of these exercises you are going to do 4 sets with 90–120 seconds (as noted next to each movement) of rest between each set before moving on to the next exercise. For example, you would finish 1 set of 5–8 bench presses, rest for 120 seconds, do another set of 5–8 reps, rest for 120 seconds, another set, rest for 120 seconds, then a final set. After resting for another 120 seconds, you will move on to seated Arnold presses and continue until you have done all the moves.

This workout should take you around an hour to finish. As always, make sure to do some dynamic stretching (active movement) before you begin, to warm up your muscles. I also recommend doing each exercise a couple of times with very light weights to prep your muscles before working with heavier weights.

The Workout

BENCH PRESS: 4 sets, 5–8 reps, 120 seconds rest

SEATED ARNOLD PRESS: 4 sets, 5–8 reps, 90 seconds rest

LATERAL PULLDOWNS (CLOSE GRIP): 4 sets, 5–8 reps, 90 seconds rest

LATERAL PULLDOWNS (WIDE GRIP): 4 sets, 5–8 reps, 90 seconds rest

STANDING TRICEP EXTENSIONS: 3 sets, 5–8 reps, 60 seconds rest

BARBELL BICEP CURLS: 3 sets, 5–8 reps, 60 seconds rest

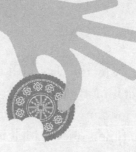

CHAPTER 5

DISCOVER YOUR ROOTS

Your identity is your most valuable possession. Protect it.

—ELASTIGIRL, *THE INCREDIBLES*

You're going to eat *that* for breakfast?" I asked my husband, judgment dripping from my lips. "You haven't even worked out today."

My husband had just gotten home from an early morning class with a treat in hand. I could see the hurt flicker across his eyes as I picked apart the doughnut he had been excited to eat just five seconds earlier. "Taylor, why do you have to pick apart all my food choices like that all the time?"

I had no idea why this was such a big deal to him. I had been trying to get him to eat healthier and bugging him about his food choices for our whole marriage; it was just who I was. He knew I was a fitness queen. I felt bad for nagging him, but how could I change who I was?

Or was it truly me? Things had been different long ago, but I had gone so far that I didn't even know when the change had begun.

Identity. It's the very soul of who we are, because it *is* who we are. It covers so much more than just our name; my own identity is not just "Taylor." Identity involves the roles we play in our day-to-day lives. It's every single bit and piece of our lives. It's the way we feel about ourselves, the words we say to ourselves, the very root of who we are.

Did you just have a desire to stand in a yoga tree pose too? Or is that just me?

When I was in my early teen years, I lost my birth certificate. Don't ask me why I was carrying around my birth certificate in my purse. I was a teen, and therefore I did not make the world's smartest choices. Of course, lo and behold, I lost my birth certificate. However, I did not realize I had done so until I got a call from the government telling me I was being flagged for identity theft. Nope, not a made-up story to add some suspense. I wish I were making this up. At this point in my life, I thought I had lost my identity. My birth certificate said everything about me—my name, my birthday, where I was born, etc. But fast-forward over a decade, and I've now come to realize that wasn't the biggest case of "identity theft" I had experienced in my life, because our identity runs so much deeper than some words on a sheet of paper.

Maybe you haven't received that no-fun call when some very important person tells you that your identity has been stolen, but at some level, we all struggle with identity, even if we don't know it yet. The world tells us who we should be by the messages it sends in the culture and in the media, and we believe it. In Gretchen Saffles's Bible study on defining identity, she says, "We have handed over who we are and who we were originally made to be to a ruthless World that etches lies, doubts and insecurity on our hearts." She goes on to say, "We don't know where to go or to whom we should report our robbery!"[1]

As you already know, we search for our worth and value inside ourselves, and because of this, we start on the Perfection Pursuit, and our search for wholeness that seems just out of reach becomes our identity—a broken identity the enemy can manipulate.

Whenever we root our identities in something we think we can achieve by our own strength, control, or something culture tells us, we are setting ourselves up to be picking those broken little pieces of our identity up off the floor, trying to stick them together with glue and wondering why we never feel whole. My own case of "identity theft" was a combination of both of those things. It was rooted in what I looked like and a desire for perfection. I believed if I controlled my body with food, exercise, and obsession, I would then achieve the perfection the world told me I needed to be the best possible, happiest, and most whole version of myself. Spending hours at the gym and only eating a certain number of calories or only "whole" and "real" types of foods became who I was. For real, if someone asked me, "Who are you, Taylor?" my gut response would be to tell them

I was a lover of fitness and vegetables. I even ate kale, and *liked it*, because I was super healthy like that.

And the biggest lie in that response is not about liking kale (because really, who does?). It was a lie about who I was and the reason I had to default to my "worldly" qualities. Who was I really? I was a wife, a daughter, a sister, a friend, a blogger, a daughter of God who is *loved* by God, and *whole* just as I was. But I wasn't able to recognize that, and I became what I now call "fitness-queen Taylor." This is the name I gave my eating-disorder personality.

Don't worry. I didn't sit around and talk to some other personality or anything. I just find it helpful to give the misguided side of yourself some kind of name or personality. It'll help us out later when we're digging into our roots.

"Fitness-queen Taylor" had it all together. She was perfect on the outside, and she was also *way* too busy working out and weighing grapes to even have time to sit down and deal with what was going on inside. She didn't have to deal with the fact that her life wasn't being lived out in a way which reflected that she *truly* believed she was a daughter of God, even though she told people she believed that. She didn't even have to deal with God because she didn't make any time for him. She knew he would make her work through the issues of her heart that she didn't want to deal with. She didn't have to deal with a misplaced sense of worth or value. But more important, she didn't have to deal with the gripping fear that quitting "fitness-queen Taylor" to uncover the true Taylor would reveal that the real Taylor was not enough, to find out that being the real Taylor would be some sort of a letdown or a failure.

I like to compare our real selves to our little-kid selves, and sometimes I refer to the person I wanted to become as "little Taylor." Our little-girl selves are who we truly are because they are not jaded by the ideals society and culture have placed on us. They are just happy. They are just joyful. They don't worry about the gym, what to eat, how to be more productive, how to have the perfect relationships or families or anything else we women try to make into identities. They just are, and they are happy doing it.

Maybe you're not a fitness queen, maybe you're "Supermom Sadie" or "Scholarly Susan" or "Successful Shelly." Or maybe you're something that doesn't start with an S. Whatever title has become your identity, we are all using them to patch up our own cases of identity theft. The underlying fear of having our own true selves not be enough is always the heart of the issue.

To some degree, we start to even wonder who our real selves are. Depending on the amount of time you've spent giving your identity over to the world, you may not even know yourself anymore. You may have even started to find joy in doing the things you think give you worth and value, telling yourself that because you enjoy what you're doing, it must be who you are. This was the case for me. I no longer knew how to separate "fitness-queen Taylor" from the true Taylor, which is why my identity became so wrapped up in the gym and my body. This happened with my job too. I started to find joy in working fourteen-hour days when I started my blog. Joy in working all day even though I neglected my husband. And so I thought I was just a workaholic and it was just the way I was designed.

Whenever I would do something "real Taylor" used to love, like having a chill, no-work, no-gym, Netflix-binge kind of day, I almost felt like I was letting the fitness queen side of me down. Maybe that's you too? When you sit and rest for a second instead of picking up every single toy your kids leave in their wake, you feel you're letting your supermom status down. Maybe when you put work away for just one hour to watch some brainless reality TV, you feel like you're letting your business self down (I feel this!), and so on and so forth. When we feel let down, or lazy, or whatever we feel, we assume we're tapping into a side of ourselves that we shouldn't be. But really, a lot of those feelings are pointing us to our *true* identity.

Sometimes we even create these identities based on what we *think* we want. But when we're deep into it, we begin to realize that what we thought we were going to get is a lie and these identities no longer serve us. However, because we've believed who we are is one way, we are too afraid to change. We are too scared to try to leave.

When we no longer understand that our false identities and our true identities are *not* the same thing, it becomes impossible to separate the two, and the only logical explanation is that they *are* the same thing. I knew that the identity I created for myself was not true, but I couldn't separate it, and I was scared to try. Deep down, I wanted out. I didn't want to be the girl who didn't eat any sugar or the girl who dead-lifted even when she felt sick as a dog, or the girl who worked from morning to night, only to stop for a gym break, but I didn't know what that looked like. I was scared to admit that I wanted to change myself. I was scared to come back to God and admit that I was living my life in a way that wasn't filling me up because I didn't trust that his way was better. I truly believed my identity was rooted in perfectly measured grapes, purse chicken, making money, and lots and lots of squats.

Do you ever say something and then, once you hear yourself, think, "What on earth am I saying, and why did I even think that?" That's what I'm thinking as I read that last sentence. I hope you're starting to identify your mistaken beliefs as well.

Girlfriend, why are we not enough just as we are? Why must we be "fitness queen," or "supermom," or "brainy businesswoman," or whatever title you've taken on for yourself? How do we stop living in fear of finding out who we truly are and start living it out and feeling confident in who that person is?

Well, we need to go back to the *very* beginning. Like, *beginning* beginning. The beginning of creation.

Genesis 1:1 says, "In the beginning God created the heavens and the earth." Right from the beginning of time, it was all about God. He was the beginning. The rest of Genesis 1 tells us that he made everything: the earth, the water, the animals, and the people. God is the great creator, the inventor, and the one who has all the ideas. Nothing exists today that was not first thought out by God. It's all about him.

And you know what Genesis 1:27 says? It says, "So God created mankind in his own image, in the image of God he created them; male and female he created them." You and I are created in the very *image* of God. We are made to be God's likeness and his image bearers. This should already give you a clue that our identities are not defined the way the world tells us to define them. We should be defining them by who we are made to imitate. We're made to imitate the creator of all things just as we are right now, right here, in this moment.

Unfortunately, culture tells us otherwise. We were originally created to reflect God's perfect character, but the world

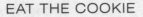

tells us *we are* the perfect character,[2] not just a reflection. It tells us *we* are the center. So many of us run around the world trying to control everything and striving for a perfection and wholeness that only God can bring. We begin to confuse who God is and who we are, and the lines become blurred. We can sometimes begin to act like *we* are God. I know this to be true in my own life. I thought I knew what was best for me, only to realize from the confines of a hospital bed, hooked up to heart monitors and eating breakfast, lunch, and dinner in a hospital room doorway, being gawked at by passersby, that I really and truly did not.

So what happened? Where did we get this God complex leading to our identity theft?

If you said, "the enemy," then *ding, ding, ding*, ten gold stars and a free virtual pedicure for you.

Second Corinthians 11:3, 14 calls the enemy deceitful and cunning and says he masquerades as an angel of light. This is *exactly* how he operated in the garden when he slithered his nasty little self up to Eve. If you thought the dark, scary path of the Perfection Pursuit was no good, the enemy is about a billion times nastier. His lie started in the garden with Eve. Genesis 3:1 says the serpent asked Eve, "Did God really say, 'You must not eat from any tree in the garden'?" He is a master of deceit, and he tried to twist God's words so Eve would question them. He wanted her to look inside herself, instead of to God, for what she thought he said. He planted seeds of doubt in her head, questioning her identity and God's words. He wanted her to take her eyes off God and find her identity within herself. This is exactly what he did with me. This is exactly what he does to you.

We may not be running around a garden anymore, but the

enemy still uses the same "Did God really say?" lie with us today. He wedges this lie between God's calling and our understanding of this divine calling.

When we listen to the lies of the enemy and begin to doubt God's truth, we begin to look inside ourselves for an identity. I didn't believe what God said about me or that his plan for my life was better than my own, so I found myself stuck looking inside myself to define who I was. Unfortunately, this always leaves us feeling miserable. And since we're made in the image of God, we're pretty poor image bearers if we're miserable with ourselves!

Adam and Eve were surrounded by perfection, yet they didn't trust God and chose to believe the serpent. Have you ever placed yourself in the "God" position, doing something you rationalized as good, only to have it end in a big mess? We've all been there. Even the first two people ended up there.

What's really interesting, and kind of funny, is that Adam and Eve chose fig leaves to cover themselves after they realized they were naked. Fig leaves aren't super common in most of the United States, so you may have never seen one, but they're tiny and are "not very user-friendly. They contain an enzyme call 'ficin,' which, when touched, can cause severe skin irritation."[3] Adam and Eve felt broken and ashamed of their choice, and they tried to use something makeshift and itchy to make coverings for themselves. You've probably never sewn fig leaves together for clothing, but you and I do something similar all the time without even realizing it.

Because we're victims of identity theft, we also live under the weight of shame—the shame of not knowing who we truly are and the shame of some foolish actions we've taken because of our misplaced sense of identity. Then we try to cover up that shame with things that irritate our very souls because they are counter to our true identity in Christ. However, we tell ourselves that these things will somehow shape us into the women we should be, making us complete. I used little bits of physical appearance, status, money, and weight to create the identity of "fitness-queen Taylor" or "hardworking-business Taylor." But we can never expect to feel whole, knowing who we are, when we counter who we are in Christ and use things that are already irritating our souls to cover the brokenness we already feel. It's not rocket science, girlfriend. Just cold, hard, logical facts.

Good news, though! The Bible tells us exactly how to get rid of this underlying shame and brokenness masquerading as identity. Psalm 34:5 says, "Those who look to him are radiant; their faces are never covered with shame." Psalm 119:5–6 says we will never be put to shame if we consider God's commands. So how do we get there? How do we take off that mask and uncover our true, full, and whole identity?

To know who *we* are, we must first know who *God* is.

There's this guy in the Bible named Moses. Ever heard of him? He was pretty cool and led tons of Israelites to freedom. But what you might not know is that he didn't feel like he could do it. He had built his identity around all his weaknesses, and when he was called to lead the people to freedom, he was *not* super psyched about it. He questioned God, asking him, "Who am I to do this?" (Exodus 3:11). God answers him in verse 14 with "I AM WHO I AM." When God identified himself as I AM WHO I AM, he meant that no matter when or where, he is always there.[4]

God doesn't just reassure Moses and tell him he can do

it. He responds to Moses's question by telling him that no matter how much Moses thinks he can't do it, God will be there. Because the story isn't really about who Moses is and his strengths and weaknesses. It's just about God being there with him, no matter what, supplying him with everything he needs to do what God calls him to do. God's identity and his abilities are in us because we are made in his image. No matter how broken we feel, no matter how irritated our souls are, we are enough just because we are made in his image. I wish I would have grasped this earlier, instead of running toward all the things I thought would give me an idea about who I truly was, but really only took me further and further away from God and who he said I was.

There arc so many other Scriptures that tell us who God is. Revelation 22:13 says he is "the Alpha and the Omega, the First and the Last, the Beginning and the End." I think of God as the "first" in the sense that God is before us in everything we do, ready to strengthen us. He is the "last" in the sense that he is always behind us, holding us up and comforting us when we're not feeling so hot.

First John 4:8 says, "Whoever does not love does not know God, because God is love." He is the very definition of love because he created love. That love should warm us like a cozy blanket by a fire or a steaming cup of hot cocoa with a lot of marshmallow action. That very love should be at the root of our hearts so that, in turn, we can place our roots in it. Our identity is rooted in God's unconditional love.

That's right. No matter how far gone you think you are, or how deep your identity theft goes, God is still there, still doing his "love thing," and still going before you and after you in everything you do. I could have never imagined that God would have stayed and loved me even when the last thing I told myself I wanted was his love, but he did. It's like those horror movies where the young teenagers are stuck in some cabin in the woods and they can't outrun their adversaries, except this is no horror movie, girlfriend. We never want to try to out-run God.

Guess what? Even if you tried, he would still love you.

No matter how much the enemy has tried to take your iden-tity from you, leaving you broken, ashamed, and not even sure of who you are, you can always come back to God. Back to his love for you. Back to knowing you are made in his image. And if he is love, and you have his image inside you, then you can love yourself just as you are. Right now.

I eventually believed this, and I stopped running away from God. Instead, I ran *to* him, and I love myself more than I could have imagined, and not in a prideful way. It's all because I understand his love for me just as I am.

There's a story in John 10:1–10 about a shepherd and his sheep. You can read the whole story, but the idea is that the shepherd leads the sheep into the pen through the gate, and the sheep know his voice. Any person who enters any other way is a "thief and a robber," and the sheep will run away from this person's voice because he is a stranger. We want to be those sheep. You're probably not too thrilled about being compared to a sheep right now, but just stick with me for a second, okay?

We have to learn to be like those cute little sheep, discern-ing the voice of God over the enemy and listening only to him. If you're anything like me, you typically listen to the voice of culture, media, or others' opinions, or maybe you even let your own feelings about yourself lead you around, trying to find who you are. First Peter 2:25 says we were like sheep going astray, but now we have returned to the Shepherd. Only when we are able to block out all that "identity noise" can we listen to the voice of God, enter his gate (Jesus), return to him, and allow *his* identity to cover us and define us.

So how do we hear his voice among the crazy lies and insecurity that the world has engraved onto our very heart and soul? If only we could be like Moses. When I read the story of God speaking to Moses through a burning bush, I get a little jealous of the guy. I mean, first he got to lead people out of slavery, which is definitely something to write home about, but he didn't have to go searching for what God wanted him to do or spend hours sitting in silence hoping that a word would come down from heaven. A bush burned and, *voilà*, God's voice and truth came to him.

Hearing the voice of God and learning to root ourselves in it is not easy, and it takes some work. But you're already reading this book, which means you are trying to hear the voice of God, and that is the very first step!

But we do need to spend time in stillness, just sitting with God. We need to ask him to send the Holy Spirit into our lives to lead us into his love and identity for us. The Holy Spirit is always with us, but I've found that when I ask him to show up, he does. You might need to get up each morning and say, "God, let me experience you today. Let me be rooted in you." Yep, say that out loud. Your significant other might look at you like you grew another head, but, hey, I'm willing to bet you'll hear God.

Learning to listen to the voice of God also applies to our thought life. Have you ever even thought about your thought life? It's a real thing, I promise. You have the power to stop and *think* about what you're thinking about, taking the time to assess if it's a cultural thought or a God thought. The only way we're going to be able to make the right assessment is if we've spent time in the Word and have asked God to speak into our lives. He won't force you to do anything. But once you take that step to reclaim your identity, girlfriend, this is no time for heels. You better go grab those running shoes, because you're in for a wild (and amazing!) ride.

THINGS TO THINK ABOUT

Before we wrap this baby up with a pretty bow, let's just press an imaginary pause button. I have a few questions for you that may help you figure out what broken pieces you're trying to stick together to make up an incorrect identity and identify who you are beyond, well, just yourself.

We talked about the "fig leaves" we use to cover up our shame and to create our identities. Knowing what your "fig leaves" are will help you be able to ask God to speak into those areas of your life. It will also give you the power to be able to recognize when you're trying to cover up. In her "Redefined" devotional, Gretchen Saffles asks the reader to consider what "fig leaves" we might be hiding behind. Let's take a look at some examples she offers, and some I have added, and identify ourselves here:[5]

- Clothes
- Status
- Money

- Social Media Followers/Social Media Likes
- Body/Appearance/Beauty
- Macros/A Specific Diet
- Accolades/Resume/Accomplishments
- Friendships/Relationships/Family
- Grades
- Possessions
- Jobs
- How "Jesus-y" you are
- Sexuality

There might be some other ones, but those are the main ones we ladies can struggle with. Just sit with that for a few seconds.

Next let's assess who we are outside of just ourselves. This is something my counselor made me do, and it allowed me to see who I was outside of my body, work, and food choices. So, for me, outside of just Taylor, I am a wife, a daughter, a sister, a blogger, a businesswoman, a friend, and now even an author! Think of all the roles you play in life. Write 'em down. Now, let's think about how we can reflect God in those roles we play in our daily lives. For example, I can pray for my husband daily, or encourage us to start a devotional book together. Or it could be as simple as being a good, kind friend, even when I feel hurt or neglected, because that is how God would react in that situation. Thinking about who we are beyond our status, body, possessions, etc., and how we can reflect God in those things, shifts our focus upward and not inward.

Our identities are not about how many days we go to the gym each week or how many grapes we do or don't eat. It's not about how good we are at our jobs, how productive we are, or how many temper tantrums our kiddos have a day.

Jeremiah 1:5 says God formed us in the womb, and he knew us. Before we were even born, he set us apart. Galatians 4:7 says we are no longer slaves to sin, but sons and heirs of God. Girl, we are *daughters* of God. That is who we are at our very core. Chosen, loved, known, and whole. No longer slaves to sin, shame, perfection, control, and identity theft.

I won't lie to you and tell you I rock at this every day. There are days when I pretty much, well, suck. Like everything I talk about in this book, this will always be a struggle because we are humans and are broken by nature. My inclination is always going to be to look to the world to tell me who I am. I have days where I see my heavier body and feel gross. Disgusting. Unworthy. Like I let "fitness-queen Taylor" down.

You know what's really cool, though? No matter how much we think we suck, or how far we've gone, or how much we can't root ourselves in a new and true identity, we're wrong. Second Corinthians 5:17 says, "Therefore, if anyone is in Christ, the new creation has come: The old has gone, the new is here!" We are *new* every day, as long as we are rooted in Christ. We are no longer stuck in our old ways. "Fitness-queen Taylor" is gone, and the new, true Taylor is being made. When I remember this, I can view my new, healthy body in a different light. I no longer feel like I am letting myself down, because I am becoming more like Christ! And this can happen for you too.

When you take a day off work, you don't need to feel lazy. You are becoming a new creation and making space for God instead of working your life away. When your kids are, you know, kids, and get a little loud, and you decide to just let them do their thing for once? You're not letting them down or being a bad mother. You're giving them and yourself space to become a new creation! I also love how Isaiah 43:18–19 says it: "Forget the former things; do not dwell on the past. See, I am doing a new thing! Now it springs up; do you not perceive it? I am making a way in the wilderness."

But, the more I am able to listen to the voice of God, replacing his identity for my own, the easier it becomes and the more I live out the free, full, and vibrant life he has planned for me, just as I am. Right here. Right now. He will make a way in the wilderness, doing a new and exciting thing in you. Transforming you away from the broken pieces of identity you thought you were and into who you were always designed to be: made in his image.

Your identity is not about what you do; it's about who made you.

Isaiah 53:5 says, "By his wounds we are healed." We are healed of our brokenness. We are healed of our shame. We are healed of identity theft. Report it to God and allow the Great I AM to define who you are.

FOR YOUR TOOLBOX

Yet to all who did receive him, to those who believed in his name, he gave the right to become children of God—children born not of natural descent, nor of human decision or a husband's will, but born of God.

—JOHN 1:12–13

But whoever is united with the Lord is one with him in spirit.

—1 CORINTHIANS 6:17

Since, then, you have been raised with Christ, set your hearts on things above, where Christ is, seated at the right hand of God. Set your minds on things above, not on earthly things. For you died, and your life is now hidden with Christ in God.

—COLOSSIANS 3:1–3

Accept one another, then, just as Christ accepted you, in order to bring praise to God.

—ROMANS 15:7

LUNCH RECIPE

"BAGEL AND LOX" EGG SALAD FOR TWO

Everything Bagel Seasoning is all the rage right now, and for good reason! It's absolutely delicious on just about anything and everything! This egg salad is mixed with smoked salmon, dill, capers, cream cheese, and Everything Bagel Seasoning so it tastes like a lox bagel without the bread! Of course, you could serve this as a sandwich, or even on a bagel if you want a little more "everything"

---

action! This egg salad uses Greek yogurt to replace mayonnaise to make it a little lighter and give it extra protein and a yummy tang!

Ingredients

3 large eggs
¼ cup plain, nonfat Greek yogurt
2 tablespoons cream cheese, softened to
  room temperature
1 tablespoon green onion, thinly sliced
2 teaspoons capers, drained
1 teaspoon Everything Bagel Seasoning
½ teaspoon fresh dill, minced
8 cherry tomatoes, halved
¼ cup smoked salmon, thinly sliced (1.5 oz)
Butter lettuce, for serving

Directions

1. Cover the eggs with about 1 inch of water and bring to a boil on high heat. Once boiling, turn off the heat (but don't remove the pot!), cover the pot, and let it sit for 12 minutes.
2. After 12 minutes, pour out the water and cover eggs with cold water. Let stand for 5 minutes.
3. Peel the cooled eggs, dice them, and place them into a large bowl. Add in the Greek yogurt, cream cheese, green onion, capers, bagel seasoning, and dill. Stir until well

combined and then stir in the tomatoes and smoked salmon.

4. Serve in lettuce leaves and devour!

PREP TIME: 10 minutes
COOK TIME: 15 minutes
SERVES: 2

Pro Tips!

1. I've made this with dairy-free yogurt as well as dairy-free cream cheese, and both work great if you can't tolerate dairy.
2. I like to make a big batch of this to have on hand for easy lunches during the week.

HEAVY BARBELL COMPLEX WORKOUT

Oh, the barbell complex. Have you ever heard of it? A barbell complex is a series of movements you perform back to back while you are holding a barbell. You complete a set number of reps per each movement before transitioning to the next movement. Seems straightforward, right? It is, but it's a lot tougher than it sounds! The barbell will never leave your hand, which really ups the intensity of the workout.

Barbell complexes are one of my favorite kinds of cardio because they are strength-based and will help increase the strength of your regular lifts and boost your endurance.

Because you are constantly moving and adding resistance, these workouts give you a big burn in a very short amount of time.

If you're short on time, you can do multiple sets of this complex as a stand-alone workout, as it will hit all your muscle groups. Or, if you really want a big finish after a regular lifting day, you can do one set at the very end of your workout to get that last little bit of energy out.

For this complex, you are going to do 5 reps of each of the movements before going onto the next movement. Remember: The barbell never leaves your hands. Although you want to move as quickly as possible, form is still always important, so you don't want to just be throwing the barbell around. Keep it controlled and feel the tension in your muscles.

We're doing only 5 reps for the workout to promote strength. If you're going for muscular endurance only, this is when we use light weights with high reps. For this complex, pick a barbell weight that makes the fifth rep tough but not totally impossible.

The Workout

BARBELL HANG CLEAN (5 REPS)

BARBELL PUSH PRESS (5 REPS)

FRONT SQUAT (5 REPS)

ALTERNATING LUNGE (5 REPS PER LEG)

BACK SQUAT (5 REPS)

If you're going to do this exercise multiple times, rest as little as you can between sets.

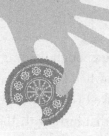

CHAPTER 6

USE SOCIAL MEDIA FOR GOOD

Never before has a generation so diligently recorded themselves accomplishing so little.

—Anonymous

My eyes fluttered open, and I rolled over to stop the buzzing of my iPhone telling me to get up and get at 'em. Before even thinking about what I was doing, the blue glare of Instagram lit up my face as I began to scroll and scroll, wondering what I had missed while I was sleeping. You can't risk missing seeing what your best friend ate for dinner last night, you know! As I scrolled, my heart raced, and I felt the nagging pressure of not being enough coming back. Would it ever stay away for longer than when I was asleep? I already felt tired, and I had only been awake two minutes!

But there was "that girl" with the "perfect body" posting about how she had already been up for three hours, gone to CrossFit, drunk a green smoothie, jade-rolled her face, and made an *epic* latte loaded with all kinds of collagen and super herbs and plants and who knows what else. I had a boring bowl of collagen-free and super herb–free bowl of oatmeal planned, and I had not yet been to the gym, drunk a green smoothie, or jade-rolled my face. I felt like I was already losing before even getting out of bed.

Everybody uses social media. Okay, scratch that. There are still people like my dad who boycott it and refuse to use it. I even asked him once if he would be my Facebook friend if he *did* have it, and he said he would *deny* my friend request just to annoy me. Dads. Can't live with them, can't be alive without one. Almost everybody uses social media. It's the way we connect with the people currently in our lives, stalk the people we *wish* we had in our lives, and creep on the people of our past lives to see what they're up to. It's where we post the pictures of our food, our workouts, our parties, our vacations, our GIFs, and almost anything else you can think of. It's all on social media for the world to see. For you and me to wake up to, scroll through, and instantly start playing the game of comparison.

Growing up, social media wasn't really a thing for me. Facebook didn't come around until I was just graduating high school, and Instagram didn't even exist until I was in my late teens. If you're in your early twenties or teens, you probably think I grew up in a cave and wrote letters on rocks to communicate with other people, don't you? Because it wasn't around, it didn't really directly play into my eating disorder. I'm grateful for that because I do not know if I would have ever recovered if the social media highlight reel would have been blowing up in my face every day like a grenade, shattering my already small self-esteem to smithereens.

But, girlfriend, without even realizing it, this is what it does to us as adults. Right now.

Social media is my world because social media is my job. Even if social media isn't your job, I'm willing to bet that you look at it, post on it, and scroll through it like it *is* your job. Do you remember the great Instagram blackout of 2019? Instagram and Facebook shut down in some parts of the world for just one day, and people freaked out. It's become such a part of our world that we almost don't even know how to function without it anymore.

Every day we scroll through photo after photo of other women with perfect bodies and perfect families, amazing jobs, and gorgeous houses, taking fabulous vacations, and looking like they rolled out of bed and got hit by the glamour truck *every single* day. We see our favorite "wellness" Instagrammers posting about their maca root salad dressing that's drizzled over a bowl with about eight hundred different vegetables, one from every color of the rainbow, sprinkled with bee pollen and goji berries, while they wash it all down with a matcha oatmilk latte.

When we look at our PB&J sandwiches, we start to feel less than. We start to feel like we can never measure up. We start to feel like we need maca root salad dressing and bowls with every vegetable known to mankind to be healthy. We need a six-pack and to get up at 4:30 for CrossFit. We need to have kids with dresses that match ours, relationships that never have any fighting, only smiling and laughing, and houses that look like they are perpetually clean. All because that's what Miss Instagram does. Plus, she gets hit by the glamour truck every day while we're just over here riding the hot-mess express.

How many times have you picked up your phone as you've read these words? Do you realize how often you subconsciously pick up your phone and mindlessly scroll? If you're anything like me, you do *not* like when your phone sends you the usage reports and it's about a billion hours that week. I am exaggerating, but you feel me.

I remember so many times I used to pick up my phone just to check Instagram, expecting to spend just a couple of minutes going through my messages, but then I would see some girl I thought had an amazing body, or a perfect family, or was on some epic vacation that I wanted to be on. Even though I knew that I shouldn't because it would start me down the road of comparison, I would click her profile anyway. This led me down this never-ending vortex of looking at her stories and then through all her photos.

When I emerged from this vortex, I had wasted at least an hour, and I would spend the rest of the day poking and prodding at my body wondering why it didn't look like hers. Or wondering why my husband and I weren't *always* smiling and laughing, or why I didn't get to go on vacations all the time and have a home that looked like it was from a magazine. I would just end up feeling like I could never measure up. And even worse, I would sometimes feel upset with God that he put me in *this* life. Why not some other fancy one like Miss Instagram's?

Social media, and therefore comparison, has become our

world. When we are spending so much time on something, taking in everything we see, read, and post, it becomes how we see the world, and therefore becomes our identity.

Social media is one of the "fig leaves" we talked about that we patch together to try to create our identities when we are afraid of truly becoming who God designed us to be. We begin to define who we are by how many followers we have, how many likes our photos get (or don't get), and by how our life is looking in comparison to the other hot Instagram girls. Social media can push you to begin to look inward, which can start us down that dark, scary Perfection Pursuit and lead us to finding worth in ourselves, our likes, and our followers. It can further push us to try to find our identity in "fig leaves" like our bodies, status, motherhood, and wealth because we see that other (happy!) people have all these things. They have it all together.

Social media was one of the very reasons I kept such tight control over my body. Remember when that trainer put my abs on Facebook? It felt good. It felt good to have people comment about how fit I looked when I posted a photo of myself. It made me feel valuable and worthy and like I was doing something right. When I started my job as a blogger or "social media influencer" as some call it, it felt good to see the number of likes on a post and to see all the comments. I would obsessively check to see how many I was getting and, if it wasn't enough, I would immediately feel negative about myself. Why am I not enough? Why is my photo not enough to get three thousand likes? Did people hate me?

Reading it on paper seems *so* silly. Why do we define who we are by how many times people click a tiny little heart or a thumbs up? I felt that if I gave up "fitness-queen Taylor," people would "heart" me less and my "thumbs up" would go down. Therefore, I wanted to control what people thought of me by only posting the best photos of my food, myself, or the dates I had with Mr. FFF.

Can I be honest with you, without judgment? Some of the things I used to post when I first started my social media accounts and blog, and was in the depths of my battle with body image and all the other issues we've talked about, weren't even reality.

The cookie recipe I posted? Although it was "healthier," I probably took one tiny bite of them to test the flavor, then spat it out because it had too many calories.

That banana bread I posted? I probably ate one bite and then made poor Mr. FFF eat all the rest because I didn't want it around me because I was afraid I would eat it.

That post I shared with a cookie the size of my head and talked about food freedom? I threw the cookie away right after I posted it.

That photo of me on a vacation looking so happy and alive? Mr. FFF and I fought right before it, and I felt more dead inside than alive.

That photo of me drinking a glass of wine? You already know I starved myself all day so that it could fit into my daily calories.

That leg workout I shared on my Instagram stories? I did it. But my body felt *so* exhausted while I was doing it because it just wanted food and rest.

That "fit" body that was shared on Facebook? It had high cholesterol, no period, and a slow thyroid because it was in starvation mode. It was far from healthy.

And on and on and on.

You're probably thinking I'm a big hypocrite and, girlfriend, back then, circa 2017, I was. I was so driven by feeling perfect and valuable, yet being so deeply afraid that the real Taylor wouldn't be seen as these things, that I didn't let you in on what I was going through. If you follow me on social media now, though, you know I've shared about working through my food issues, my mental health issues, and my actual health issues. I actually eat everything I post. I go to yoga usually, but not if I'm feeling bad. Heck, at the time of writing this, it's been nine months since I've lifted a weight because I am 100 percent committed to healing my body. I probably still don't post my arguments with Mr. FFF, but I no longer post fake happy photos of us, and I am real about our marriage having harder moments. I don't feel dead inside. I feel *alive*.

We both know Instagram isn't reality. And as a social media influencer myself, I'm just here to keep it real and shed some light on it. There are *many* people on social media who are still posting fake things. They're still posting food they do not eat, workouts they did even though they were exhausted, and how healthy they are when they too are in a body that is not so healthy on the inside. There are people posting about their perfect-looking homes, but not about the strife inside that home. Or their adorable little children who are angels, but you don't see the many meltdowns it took for them to take the photo, and so on and so forth.

Instagram is just the highlight reel of everyone's life. I know you have been told this a million times, but it can still be *so* hard for us to remember this. I am not saying everyone is like this, I just want you to remember that when you're looking through your feed, you're not seeing all the moments of everyone else's life. You're not seeing the thoughts that drive them to look a certain way or do a certain thing, and from my own experience and those of fellow social media influencers, they're not always done from a healthy mindset.

And for what? When I stumbled on our chapter's opening quotation, "Never before has a generation so diligently recorded themselves accomplishing so little," it hit me like a loaf of gluten-free bread from the '90s. You totally know that the early versions of gluten-free bread were like rocks. My dad used to have to eat it, and I called it "alien bread." It's definitely come a long way since then.

Did you kind of get hit in the gut when you read that quotation too? I never really realized this truth until I read that statement. Back in the day, when people accomplished something, you would only hear about them if they were written down. You didn't have people posting about their everyday lives and letting other people peer in on them. Only important discoveries or findings were recorded.

But with social media, we record ourselves eating breakfast, we record ourselves at the gym, we record what macros we are eating to get the perfect six-pack, our beautiful vacations, or our kids' perfect grades. There isn't anything wrong with wanting to post about things that are important to you on social media—it is my job after all, and I think posting about food is pretty awesome. But when we start seeing these things as accomplishments, and start getting validation from people who don't know us, that is when things start to ride the crazy train, and we start to seek out our identity and worth in social media.

Have you ever wondered what God has to say about social media? I mean, there aren't any verses directly pointing to social media, and Moses wasn't out there taking selfies with the Israelites or posting perfectly styled pictures of the manna that fell from heaven. However, I did a little digging and found some relevant Scripture I think will really help us out when we start getting into the deadly trap of comparison.

Remember that the enemy "prowls around like a roaring lion looking for someone to devour" (1 Peter 5:8), and, girlfriend, social media is one of the major ways he is eating us up today. All the issues we have been talking about—perfection, worth, identity, fear, and control—can stem from the comparison we feel when we scroll through social media.

I am sure some wise old grandma once said to you, "Comparison is the thief of joy," and you just rolled your eyes. But it's really true. I was always much less happy in my own body, with my number of likes, or the growth of my blog when I compared it to what I saw on Instagram. I was also a lot further away from God when I was using Instagram in the wrong way and only as a means to get validation and grow my "following." I was busier focusing on gaining the love of other people than I was on realizing I was already wrapped up in God's love. That cozy-fuzzy-blanket-lots-of-marshmallows-in-the-hot-chocolate kinda love.

I imagine you know exactly how it feels not to be satisfied with your life when you're comparing it to what you see on social media. I imagine the enemy loves the invention of social media because he doesn't even need to prowl around and look for people to devour! We are all there, faces lit up with the creepy blue glow, eyeballs glued to the screen, feeling insecure. When the enemy senses those insecurities and doubts, he is able to devour us so much more easily. He won't skip a beat. As soon as you open an app and even the tiniest bit of jealousy, comparison, or insecurity enters your pretty little head, he will jump on it and send you right down the dark, scary Perfection Pursuit.

Not only does comparison steal our joy, it also doesn't allow us to love other people well. When we are comparing ourselves to other people, we are not seeing them as the person God designed—beautiful and unique. We are only seeing a person to measure up to and compete with. Comparison turns our focus back inward instead of upward, and totally zaps our ability to love and accept others. It forces us to feel bad about ourselves, and the only way to feel better about our lives is to tear someone else down so we can feel better than them.

The comparison trap doesn't allow us to recognize that we are all part of the body of Christ, and we all have different jobs to do. Romans 12:4–5 says, "Just as each of us has one body with many members, and these members do not all have the same function, so in Christ we, though many, form one body, and each member belongs to all the others." You don't feel bad about your arm because it can't do the same thing as your leg, right? But this is what we do when we compare ourselves to others. We are unable to recognize that they have different strengths that they bring to the body of Christ, just as we have strengths the body of Christ needs that they don't have. We need to love them for what they bring to the table instead of trying to pull their chair out from under them.

God doesn't compare us with the other women in the world. He already knows he made us all different and all with a different purpose and strength, and this is something I wish I would have known and trusted God with sooner in my life. The only person God compares us to is to the woman he wants us to be. The woman who can love others well and love herself well. The woman who knows we all have a job and is secure in the fact she can't do *all* the jobs, but she can do *her* job.

Comparing ourselves to others is also like telling God he made a mistake. I absolutely love Romans 9:20–21 because it just hits this point so well. It says, "But who are you, a human being, to talk back to God? 'Shall what is formed say to the one who formed it, "Why did you make me likes this?"' Does not the potter have the right to make out of the same lump of clay some pottery for special purposes and some for common use?" As John Piper puts it, "God is the Potter, and we are his pots. Therefore, He decides what is right and fitting for our lives."[1] It's not up to us to decide what we look like or what our abilities are. God doesn't make mistakes, and we have no right to question him!

Whenever we complain that she has nicer arms, a better job, more-controlled kids, or whatever it is, we are telling God he made us wrong. This is something I *really* wrestled with God over for almost a decade. I was constantly talking back to God and telling him he made a mistake in how he made me when I was desperately trying to look like other women or wishing I had their success or their life. And that constant arguing against his purpose for me put a wedge between us because I couldn't just sit in his love and trust that he made me exactly how I should be made.

The Bible tells us we are fearfully and wonderfully made. It doesn't tell us we are made wrong. Instead of talking back to God, why don't we thank God for making us all a part of his body and all with different abilities? We can thank him that there are women doing the things we can't, and that we are able to do the things they can't. When I was able to have this mindset shift and sit at God's feet, living in his love and trusting him, it was like that wedge slowly disappeared, and my walk with him grew closer.

Finally, the last problem with comparison is that it breeds more comparison. When we compare ourselves to another woman, and then do everything we can to live up to her "perfection," we then become part of the comparison problem. When I compared myself to other "perfect" bodies, and then made my body fit into that ideal, I know I became a problem for other women. Other women would compare themselves with my body and feel like they were not enough. Without even realizing it, the comparison game I played led other beautiful women down the Perfection Pursuit.

So, how do we prevent this? I could tell you to never open social media again, but then I'd be taking a ride back into "hypocrite Taylor" land because social media is my job, and I know I won't just leave it behind. Social media can be great, but we have to learn how to be alert and of sober mind (1 Peter 5:8) so we can safeguard our minds from cracks that allow the enemy to slip in.

Second Corinthians 10:12 says, "We do not dare to classify or compare ourselves with some who commend themselves. When they measure themselves by themselves and compare themselves with themselves, they are not wise." Look! There was no social media in biblical times, but it already talked about the comparison trap. And it says those people who compare themselves with others are not wise. The people you follow who make you feel like not enough if you don't drink a turmeric matcha smoothie or count macros or have a more perfect house are not wise. They are looking inward and commending themselves for what *they* can do.

We talked about looking inward, and it only leads to insecurity, anxiety, fear, and doubt. First Chronicles 16:11 tells us to seek the Lord! We should not be seeking what others are, have, or do, or comparing ourselves to others. When we seek the Lord first, we find our worth, value, and security, and this allows us to become stronger so we can safeguard against the ways the enemy uses social media to make us feel small.

Social media is, by definition, social. It's where we chat with our friends and keep up with what is going on in their lives. However, with the millions of people on social media, it's easy to think we have a ton of "friends," but in reality we have a ton of people who don't truly know us or care about us. We get up every day and try to make those people think we are super cool by the things we post. And all those people are doing the same thing. We're all on this hamster wheel of craziness trying to impress our "friends" and are left feeling like we never measure up. Proverbs 18:24 says, "One who has unreliable friends soon comes to ruin, but there is a friend who sticks closer than a brother." If one who has unreliable friends soon comes to ruin, and we're constantly trying to impress our fake social media friends, how can we *not* expect it to come to ruin? In this scenario, ruin doesn't have to be some life-shattering, horrible thing that happens to you. When we allow the enemy to feed off our insecurity and doubts, causing us to chase perfection, control, and comparison, we are ruining ourselves. We are not living out our true selves and living the lives God has for us, all because we want to please some fake friends on the internet.

Just so we're clear, I know not all our friends on the internet are fake. I talk to my real and true friends there all the time. But, do you really know all the people who are liking your photos? "Bad company corrupts good character" (1 Corinthians 15:33), and if the company we are keeping are the very people who make us doubt our worth and doubt what God says about us, then our good character is going to be corrupted. Being corrupt doesn't mean we're going to start some offshore bank account and start money laundering (I watch way too much TV, can you tell?), but we can become corrupt by thinking we are the center of everything and must perform so we can be accepted. Corrupt thinking is measuring our worth and value by how many likes we have, or how our body, marriage, kids, work, or anything else stacks up against the people we see in our feeds. So where does it end and how does it stop? Can we use social media for good? I am here to tell you Y-E-S! But it's going to take some real intentionality and a lot of thinking before you post.

There is so much good to be said on social media. Among the sea of false friends, we can make some amazing connections. I've met some of my best friends on the internet. Although, if you ask Mr. FFF, I can't call them "friends" because some of them I've met once and some of them never! But social media has opened doors for us to connect with people all over the world. It has given us the ability to share our lives with family and friends far away so we don't lose touch. We're even able to share the gospel message of truth and point people to Jesus. But none of this is going to happen if you and I are using it in the wrong way.

Here's a little background about how I fell into social media. When I first got married, I was managing a dental office. Teeth are great and necessary and all, but they are not my passion. When I got married and realized I needed to learn to cook and keep someone else alive, I started creating recipes. My husband told me to start a blog, and I did, thinking just my mom would read it. She did, of course. But after a year or so, many other people started reading it! This was totally unexpected, but I fell in love with blogging and social media and worked very hard to quit my job and do it full time. And God provided the ability for me to do that. I will say I started using social media for the wrong reasons—to promote my brand and, honestly, to promote an unhealthy, obsessive way of living. I've now come to realize that while I can't avoid social media, I no longer have to use it in this way. I can (and do!) use it promote true health and freedom in Jesus Christ. As I like to say, social media has now let my mess become my message! He can do that for you too!

I imagine not all of you are bloggers, so how do you use it for good even if it's not your job? We need to be testing our own actions, so we can take pride in ourselves and not compare ourselves to each other (Galatians 6:4). What this looks like for me is really stopping to think before I post. What am I saying in a caption? Is it something I truly believe? Is this something that could be a trigger for someone else, making them feel less than, unworthy, or unvaluable. How about that picture I am about to share? Why am I posting it? Is it because I look like I have it all figured out? Did I take thirty-two selfies before posting one so I would look just right?

If you want to get all biblical, we can look to Galatians 1:10, which says, "Am I now trying to win the approval of human beings, or of God? Or am I trying to please people? If I were still trying to please people, I would not be a servant of Christ." I am not saying you're not a Christian if you find you're a little self-focused, but this verse hit me in the gut and really challenged me to ask myself a lot of questions about the things I share across social media.

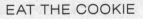

The temptation with social media is to post and move on. But while you may move on, the post stays forever stuck in the feed. People can always look at it, read it, and compare themselves to it. Whether you have twelve or one thousand followers, people are still reading what you post, wondering how you spend your time, and looking at your highlight reel because we all have influence. You are an influencer even if that's not how you make money. It takes real intentionality to think through each post, but it's the only way we're going to bring social media around to be an influence for good. Plus, when we intentionally think through our posts, we can take pride in knowing we've done our part to stop the comparison trap.

If you think through your post while asking yourself some tough questions, and you find that there is an inkling you might be posting something for praise, or you've been finding your worth in hearts or thumbs up, Philippians 2:3 can be super helpful. It says, "Do nothing out of selfish ambition or vain conceit. Rather, in humility value others above yourselves."

Once you've determined why you are posting, shift your focus to how you are posting. How can I turn this caption or photo around to make people feel better about themselves instead of tearing themselves down? Maybe that means some things never get posted. Maybe that means you post the first selfie you take, even if it is a little less than perfect. Maybe that means you take a picture of what you really ate, or maybe that means you're honest about some struggles you're having with your family. Whatever it is, when we shift our perspective to building others up instead of building ourselves up, that is when social media is amazing.

Another way we can get out of the crazy comparison cycle is by following Romans 12:15, which says, "Rejoice with those who rejoice; mourn with those who mourn." When we see a woman who is having a win and sharing it, we can be happy for her. We can build her up instead of trying to mentally tear her down so we feel better about ourselves. We can choose to rejoice for her and that she is tuning in to God's design for her life. While we see less mourning on social media, when we do see someone being vulnerable and sharing a sad part of her life, we can build her up and encourage her to keep going. We can use opportunities like these to realize everyone does not have it all together, so we don't have to have it all together either.

When we do all these things, that is when we will be able to stay in our lanes, to quit comparing, to seek our worth first in God, and to use social media for the amazing thing it can be.

FOR YOUR TOOLBOX

Do not conform to the pattern of this world, but be transformed by the renewing of your mind. Then you will be able to test and approve what God's will is—his good, pleasing and perfect will.

—ROMANS 12:2

Do not let any unwholesome talk come out of your mouths, but only what is helpful for building others up according to their needs, that it may benefit those who listen.

—EPHESIANS 4:29

"I have the right to do anything," you say—but not everything is beneficial. "I have the right to do anything"—but not everything is constructive.

—1 Corinthians 10:23

LUNCH RECIPE

MIDDLE EASTERN CHICKEN WRAPS

Middle Eastern flavors are one of our favorites! These chicken wraps are flavored with bold spices and then grilled for a smoky, charred taste. Fresh, crisp cucumbers and tomatoes, along with bursts of mint and cilantro, balance all the smoky, spicy flavors in a delicious and addictive way. This is the perfect work lunch that is packed with protein to keep you full!

Ingredients

For the chicken
2 tablespoons tomato paste
1/2 teaspoon garlic, minced
1/2 teaspoon smoked paprika
1/4 teaspoon cumin
1/4 teaspoon salt
1/8 teaspoon cinnamon
Pinch of allspice
Pinch of pepper

---

1 teaspoon olive oil

½ lb boneless, skinless chicken breast, cubed

For the wraps

¼ cup hummus

2 tablespoons tahini

2 teaspoons fresh lemon juice

4 (8-inch) tortillas

4 cups lettuce, shredded

1 ⅓ cups cucumber, finely chopped (1 large cucumber)

1 cup Roma tomato, finely chopped (2 small tomatoes)

2 tablespoons fresh mint, minced

2 tablespoons cilantro, minced

Pinch of salt

Directions

1. In a medium bowl, mix together all the chicken ingredients—except the chicken—until well combined. Add in the cubed chicken and stir to coat in the tomato mixture. Cover and refrigerate at least 1 hour or overnight.

2. Once marinated, heat your grill to medium heat and skewer the chicken onto two skewers. Cook until no longer pink inside, about 8–10 minutes, rotating about ever 2–3 minutes.

3. While the chicken cooks, mix together the hummus, tahini, and lemon juice until a thick

paste forms. Divide between the 4 tortillas and spread all over them. Top each tortilla with 1/4 of the lettuce, 1/4 of the cucumber, 1/4 of the tomato, 1/4 of the mint, and 1/4 of the cilantro. Sprinkle with a pinch of salt.

4. Divide the chicken between the tortillas, and wrap up tightly.

5. Devour!

PREP TIME: 20 minutes
COOK TIME: 10 minutes
MARINATING TIME: at least 1 hour
SERVES: 4

Pro Tips!

1. I like to make the chicken and hummus mixtures ahead of time, and then just assemble the wraps as I need them, or the night before if you're bringing them to work.

2. If you do not want to use the tahini, you can use more hummus. I just love the richness of flavor you get from the tahini!

3. If you use bamboo skewers, remember to soak them in water for at least an hour before skewering or they will catch on fire on the grill!

MY FAVORITE CARDIO FINISHER

Cardio finishers are a great way to tack a little bit of cardio onto the end of a weight-based workout! They are one of my favorite ways to end my training, and I add a cardio finisher to almost all my weight-training workouts.

Cardio finishers can be brutal. You are at the end of your workout, and you're tired. You're hungry, and you're ready to throw in the towel. But you probably have a *little* bit more in you to burn, and this last bit will get you stronger and make you feel amazing. This is the job of the workout finisher.

This cardio finisher is a 2–3 round workout with 5 different exercises per round. It starts with 15 burpees to really get your heart rate going and your body burning. After you've completed 15 burpees, you will immediately pick up a medium-weight kettlebell and do 20 kettlebell swings. Remember to watch your form and keep your abs tight and tailbone tucked. Drive the kettlebell forward and up using your glutes. Doing these things will prevent injury. After you've done the swings, immediately drop to the ground and do pushups. You can have your knees on the ground or lifted depending on your strength. Do pushups to failure, which means you literally fail and fall to the ground on the last one. You will then do 10 "man makers." These are *very* tough, so if you cannot use any weight, that is perfectly okay. As always, listen to your body. Finally, you will put the weights aside and perform 20 mountain climbers per leg. You will then rest for 1 minute and repeat the circuit a total of 2–3 times. This should take around 10–15 minutes. Aim to get faster every time you do it!

EAT THE COOKIE

The Workout

15 BURPEES

20 KETTLEBELL SWINGS

PUSHUPS TO FAILURE

10 MAN MAKERS

20 MOUNTAIN CLIMBERS (PER LEG)

Rest 1 minute. Repeat a total of 3 times.

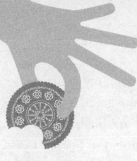

CHAPTER 7

FEEL THE FEAR AND DO IT ANYWAY

Feel the fear and do it anyway.

—MY DAD

The tour bus rolled to a stop outside our bed-and-breakfast, and my husband and I got off. Our bellies were full of chocolate and sandwiches and sausages and other "unhealthy" things we had sampled during our trip to a little German town. We waddled back up the driveway, my thoughts overflowing with anxiety. What had I done to my body today? I had eaten so much. I was probably going to gain fifty pounds over this weekend, I could just feel it. Then my husband would no longer find me attractive, and I would no longer be Taylor—the lies

145

kept flitting through my brain. As we walked into the bed-and-breakfast, we were greeted with a glass of port and a chocolate tart. It smelled and looked delicious, and I wanted it. I was scared that I wanted it. Scared to eat it. I knew I had to push those lies aside, and I grabbed that chocolate tart. It was rich, creamy, and purely soul satisfying.

A couple of days after returning from this weekend getaway, I jumped on the scale expecting to see a huge increase. My palms were sweaty, and my mind was racing. What would I do if I had gained weight? Would all the thoughts I had come true? I looked down at the scale as it beeped back at me.

Nothing. I hadn't even gained an ounce.

All that worrying for nothing.

If I had a penny for every time my dad has told me to feel the fear and do it anyway, I would be a millionaire. If I also had a penny for every time I resisted the "do it anyway" part because the fear was too great, I would be a billionaire. I probably need to tattoo it onto my forehead so I remember it. It's also the phrase that has played over and over again in my mind as I finally started to heal.

Girlfriend, we have done some *work*. We have walked down the scary path of the Perfection Pursuit. We've uncovered some possible judgments of other people that may be holding us back. We've waded way down into the deep end of our inner souls and discovered some brokenness we've tried to stick back together to make our identities. We've figured out some areas where we're searching for perfection, only to find out that achieving that "perfection" hasn't satisfied us. You know what's next in our story? Freedom. But you know what freedom requires? Stepping out into the unknown.

And that is *scary*.

I don't know about you, but I think I was a lot less afraid of the unknown as a child. When I was recovering from anorexia when I was only thirteen, I remember choosing to eat the chocolate cake over the chicken because it was scary and because I wanted to overcome it. The warrior-princess spirit was in little Taylor, and she was ready for battle. Maybe you were not overcoming a fear of chocolate cake over chicken when you were a kid, but something tells me you were a lot more fearless as a kid too. We're more comfortable with the uncomfortable when we're little tykes just learning about and challenging the things we know.

But then we grow up.

We become uncomfortable with the uncomfortable.

We get set in our habits.

We start to believe that all the thoughts that pass through our head in a given day are actually true.

We form new identities that feel overpowering.

We can do all this hard work of digging deep and uncovering the roots of our issues, but we're never going to be able to step out and choose faith over fear if we don't feel that fear and do it anyway. This was my life for so many years. I knew in my heart what I needed to do to become free from my addiction to the perfect body and the bondage that control, food, and body image had over me, but I just wasn't able to take that first step. I found myself waking up every single day saying, "Today will be the day. Today is the day when I venture out into the unknown, take back my life, and step into the big life God has planned for me."

And I'd fail before breakfast.

I would start to scroll through social media as soon as my eyes opened, which immediately led me to already feel bad about myself. I would end up feeling so frustrated that my life didn't measure up that I'd be angry with God for not planting me into another life, then I'd skip my morning devotionals. I would keep feeling bad about myself until I was back on the Perfection Pursuit, then I would start trying to control everything so I could start to feel better than whatever made me feel bad that day. I'd immediately begin to plan what I would eat that day instead of allowing my actual hunger to lead me and begin the ever-so-boring, calorie-counting repetition that played over and over in my head like a disc with a scratch on it. And this was all before breakfast! I'd end my day feeling exhausted, hopeless, and frustrated with God because of the wedge I felt in our relationship. I had the best intentions when my feet hit the floor, but then something happened, and it was like I never set those intentions. Can you relate?

I remember crying so many nights, wondering why that same little Taylor who chose chocolate cake over chicken wasn't in my life anymore. I knew it was God who gave little Taylor the power to choose those things, and I wondered why he wasn't showing his power for big Taylor. I felt stuck, and I didn't know why. Maybe you're not stuck in the endless cycle of body-image and food obsession, but maybe you're stuck in the cycle of finding your worth in your relationships or trying to get validation from people based on your ability to be the boss at work. Maybe you still equate the way your children behave with your worth and ability to be a good mom. Whatever it is, we get stuck in our habits, and we are too afraid to test the waters of breaking out of them. We don't want to even try to take that first step because there is just too much scary darkness swirling around when we do.

As alone as you feel in that moment, you're not. All the other people in the universe are feeling the fear and not wanting to do it anyway right along with you. Guess what? There were even people in the Bible who were in the same boat! We see this in Exodus, when the Israelites are wandering around and complaining, wanting to go back to their old bondage. They're getting uncomfortable with the unknown and they want to get back to the comfort of knowing what is going to happen next. They were being led by a dude who literally heard God speaking out of a burning bush, yet they questioned and doubted him and wanted to turn right back around.

We're those Israelites today. I was one of those Israelites for *so* long, calling out and complaining to God and wondering why he just kept me letting me wander. We complain and are scared to take that step of moving forward into the unknown. We stay walled up in our self-made fear fortress, unwilling to open the door and see what happens if we respond to the knock of God's freedom because it might mess up our lives and change our identities and, therefore, our perceived sense of our worth.

Just when the Israelites were about to throw in the manna and turn right back around, they turned the corner and there was Elim. Exodus 15:27 says Elim had twelve springs and seventy palm trees! I don't know about you, but I'm thinking Elim sounds pretty amazing. Can you imagine being an Israelite? You had just been wandering through a *desert* for a very long time, and you come across that? Cue that "Hallelujah Chorus"!

Elim was always coming up, and God knew that. But the Israelites did not. They probably assumed God was going to let them wander around the desert forever and ever because they, like us, thought they had all the facts. They didn't want to walk out into the uncomfortable unknown because that was scary and insecure. Even though their old life of bondage and slavery was not something they enjoyed at all, they wanted to go back because it was comfortable. But when they trusted God and took that step, they came to Elim, the land with palm trees and springs of water that would renew their tired, famished, and dehydrated bodies. They came to a land that gave them life and freedom from the oppression of their old life under the reign of Pharaoh.

This is me. This is you. We get so comfortable with the lies we believe and the patterns we create that thinking about doing life any other way, even if it could possibly be *better*, is pretty darn scary.

When I read the story of Elim, it hit me. I realized I had known what to do all along, but I was just too afraid to make that first step. And truth be told, it hit me that I didn't trust God. The Israelites were scared, but they followed God's leading and it took them to a place of comfort and freedom. I had always told myself the story of the Israelites wandering around the desert and told myself that this season of body-image obsession was just my desert and I had to go through it. I assumed that one day, if I just kept walking through my desert, I would come out the other side.

I never wanted to acknowledge that in the story of Elim, the Israelites had to *choose* discomfort to find comfort. I was much safer in my fear fortress, and you probably feel the same way. But, girlfriend, we can only find true happiness and freedom when we break down the fortress one brick at a time, no matter how uncomfortable it is. We have to get comfortable with the uncomfortable. If I would not have decided to choose discomfort and bank on the fact that God has it figured out, I would not be writing this book today. My mess would not have become my message, and I would have gone through all this hardship for nothing. Now it can be used for good. That is *my* Elim.

Like we talked about earlier, when we do some digging and find out we're not living in our pretty, Pinterest-perfect house like we thought, and we're actually living in a cold, dark fear fortress, this can point us to our need for God. I say "can" because sometimes we get so wrapped up in the fear of the unknown that we don't realize we're walled up. In that scenario, we are not able to recognize our need for God.

For many years in my life I thought I was "mostly free." I didn't really see my lifestyle as a problem because I told myself I was just being healthy, and there is nothing wrong with that. However, after much digging, I had to come to the realization that "being healthy" had begun to rule my life and I wasn't living in a way I actually wanted or that showed I trusted God. I realized I was truly walled up in a fear fortress that I didn't even know existed.

Once we do that digging into our soul and uncover the areas where we are walled up in fear, we can welcome that fear in our lives and allow it to point us to a greater need. Although we think we are superwomen, *hear us roar*, we don't have the tools to break down our own fear fortresses. When we feel our inner Bob the Builder trying to build up those walls, and we're in a healthy place of recognizing this happening, we can look to Jesus to hand us the tools to break down the walls. It's not easy, and it won't happen overnight. But the first step is recognizing this area in your life. Slowly but surely, you'll allow yourself to step out in faith, trust God, and get a little uncomfortable.

Think of yourself as a fairy-tale princess who is locked up and being guarded by a big, evil, fire-breathing dragon. The dragon is the enemy in this story. But isn't there always a handsome prince who comes to save the princess? This is Jesus. He's coming on his pretty white horse to save you.

But only if you take his hand and trust him.

Have you ever heard of "future tripping"? When I first heard the term, I thought it was some kind of "woo-woo Earth Momma" kind of thing. Then I heard the description. You trip yourself out over what *could* happen in the future, and you end up going down this long, dark, scary hole. I used to worry that if I had one day when I overate or didn't exercise, the next day I would be a balloon. And if I was a balloon, I would be ugly. If I was ugly, my husband would leave me. If my husband left me, I would die alone because I would be ugly and no one would want to be with me. Also, if I was overweight, I would no longer be "fitness-queen Taylor," so who would I be? Would I just be average? I just could not handle average.

Writing that future trip down now and seeing how my thought process used to be makes it seem so silly. But it's something I used to get an A+, gold medal, *and* a gold star in. I *aced* future tripping. Maybe your process looks something like, "If I don't climb my way to the top of the corporate ladder and become a CEO, people will view me as just a dumb girl. If I am just a dumb girl, then no one will respect me or want to be friends with me. If no one respects me or wants to be my friend, I will end up friendless and flipping burgers for the rest of my life." That might be a slight exaggeration, but, girlfriend, we perfectionists are really good at this future tripping thing.

Future tripping led me to build my fear fortress. When we

don't trust God with the future, we think all the things we are trying to achieve will not happen.

We won't be perfect.

If we're not perfect, we're not valuable.

Our broken identities become threatened.

We'll get on an out-of-control tailspin and we won't be able to stop.

All of this because of some false beliefs. We're going to talk more about how we fall into false thought patterns in the next chapter, but you get my point. When we decide what the outcomes of choosing faith over fear and stepping out of our tiny little comfort zones are before we even begin, we won't ever do it. The enemy has programmed our brains to determine the worst possible situation. I never once thought, "If I eat this cookie, it will not do one thing to me except make me happy because I like cookies." And, if I am happy, then I am able to love myself more. And if I am able to love myself, then I can love my husband and my family and friends better. Then I will have a long, happy life where I enjoy cookies and where people enjoy being around me, and I will not die alone. That kind of future tripping would be helpful, not hurtful. But you and I both know we just do not think like that.

I once listened to a podcast[1] that talked about future tripping, but then connected it to Romans 12:2; "Do not conform to the pattern of this world, but be transformed by the renewing of your mind. Then you will be able to test and approve what God's will is—his good, pleasing and perfect will." When we future trip in a hurtful way, we are conforming to what the enemy (or the world) wants us to believe. When we do this, we do not tap into the transformational power we have when we are able to separate our untrue thoughts from God's will for our lives.

This is why I lived in my pit of lies for so long, believing what the enemy said about me and calling out to God to help me, but never feeling like he did. I was so busy thinking of all the bad things that were going to happen to me that it left no room in my brain to even toy with the idea of trusting that God would work out my future in an entirely different way.

When we're able to test our thoughts and see if they are from God or from the world, our future tripping changes. Sure, we may think all those silly thoughts, like eating a cookie will turn me into a friendless balloon overnight, but we are able to trust God is with us every step of the way. And, if it is his will for unpleasant or uncomfortable things to happen, he will renew our minds to be able to handle that situation. We just must take that uncomfortable step and trust him one step at a time. Until we do this, we are not able to step out and begin to heal.

If you don't trust that this is going to be the case, look at 2 Timothy 1:7. It says, "For the Spirit God gave us does not make us timid, but gives us power, love and self-discipline." Read that again slowly. Power! God's Spirit living in us gives us power. We *are* superhero women when we allow the Spirit of God to renew our minds, because we will then get power. The power to be able to face our fear and take a step. The power to accept the outcomes. The power to be free, whole, and happy. If we're feeling too scared to take a step, we can be sure we are not operating in the power God wants to give us. I came to realize that little Taylor, who chose the chocolate cake over the chicken, had been operating in this power, and big Taylor had not been.

Being able to trust God to renew our minds and give us the

power to handle whatever happens when we walk out into the unknown isn't easy, and it doesn't just happen. We *have* to be intentional about it, and we have to actually start taking those scary steps. Even if they are baby steps, we have to take them. Taking a baby step while shaking with fear is better than just standing in one place while shaking with fear.

For me, that was slowly starting to increase my calories. Then, it was starting to miss a workout day just because. Not because I was sick or on vacation, just because. This extended into my workaholic tendencies with my job too. I slowly started working and sleeping regular hours. I started making time for devotionals. Then I started to take full days off! The more I did this, the less scary it became, and the more freedom I tasted, the more freedom I wanted. Also, the more I did this, I was able to see that my version of future tripping was totally and completely false. The things I told myself would happen did not happen. I was able to separate those as false fears and lies from the enemy.

Take a second to stop here and think of some baby steps you could take. Could you stop being a helicopter mom and let your kids make their own choices to stop tying your worth to having a perfect family? Could you maybe go out with friends for a night instead of studying a billion hours? I'm not saying just throw all your responsibilities out the window and go crazy, but where are you future tripping? These are the areas that need a couple of baby steps.

Now, I'm going to be real with you. It's not going to be flowers and açai bowls and rainbows when you do this. Fear is fear for a reason. But remember, it's False Evidence Appearing Real, which aligns with future tripping. Future tripping is our fearful thoughts appearing real. You're going to feel like the

Israelites and want to turn right back around and go back to your comfortable fear fortress. You might not trust that God will renew your mind at first, but as you take a half of a baby step forward, you'll slowly believe it.

STRATEGIES TO FEEL THE FEAR AND DO IT ANYWAY

If you read this and decided you wanted a piece of that power so you just took a step out and started doing the scary, I want to be you when I grow up. But, alas, I was not able to "just do it," and I am willing to bet you might be more inclined to be like me. You might need some helpful strategies in place that allow you to slowly step into the unknown and take hold of the power that leads to healing. I took small, tiny baby steps for almost ten years, so I think I have a little bit of insight into this and want to give you the scoop.

Strategy One: Go Back to Your Life Checkin'
Remember the "life check" we talked about earlier? Not only do those checks help you identify when you are living in fear, but doing them will also help you take that step out, choosing faith over fear. When we can identify if something is causing us to just exist instead of thrive, we can come to the conclusion that if we want to thrive, we need to do the opposite of what we are currently doing. "Do" is an action word. Stepping out and doing the scary thing is the action.

So for me, when I used to go out for dinner and start to become fearful of what I would eat and immediately try to find what I thought would be the lowest-calorie option, I needed to press pause. I needed to ask myself, "Is this boring salad with dry chicken and dressing on the side, which I might not even use because I will somehow convince myself I love the taste of plain lettuce, causing me to thrive?" I know myself, and I know that while I would feel superior because I chose to eat sad, naked leaves, I would not be present in the conversation with my husband because of all the thoughts and feelings I was having about the awesome-looking burger I *really* wanted. That is *not* thriving.

The same goes for when I am feeling the need to work, work, work from the time I get out of bed to the time I get back into it. I need to ask myself if I am thriving. I know the answer would be no, because I'll be ignoring my husband, ignoring my own needs, and feeling exhausted, overwhelmed, and anxious.

Life is too short to convince yourself you like plain lettuce. You, my friend, are not a rabbit.

Strategy Two: Find an Accountability Person

Sometimes this strategy can actually be scarier than taking a step toward freedom and away from bondage because it requires us to get personal—to get deep and vulnerable with someone. Since culture praises a lot of the issues we women struggle with these days—fitting a particular body ideal, attaining supermom status, or being workaholics or brainiacs—it can be really hard for people to know there is something deeper going on.

My husband knew I was obsessed with working out and food, since it's pretty hard to hide that kind of issue, but he didn't know how deeply rooted it was. He didn't know I had turned "fitness-queen Taylor" into my identity and that I didn't feel worthy or valuable if I did something to let her down. So I had to tell him. I had to tell him I felt the need to be skinny because I still wanted praise from people and attention from other men, even though I was so happily married to him and madly in love. It was something I needed to feel valued and worthy, and that sucks to tell your husband. It hurt him, and it hurt me to open up about it. But once I was open with him, he was able to come alongside me and encourage me. He was able to help me perform those life checks when he saw I was struggling. He would encourage me and let me know when I was being more fun and free, even if I felt like I was letting "fitness-queen Taylor" down or spiraling out of control.

What is even more awesome is that when I told him more about what was going on in my brain, he was more open and honest with things he had been struggling with. This allowed our relationship to be deeper as we were able to help each other and take steps together. Sometimes our hang-ups become our handles that open doors to deeper connection.

My family always knew I was struggling as well because they knew me before I started walking down the Perfection Pursuit, so they could see the change in me. I know it was incredibly hard for them to see me living a life without the carefree and happy Taylor they knew lived inside of me. The way my mom looked at me sometimes with utter sadness and a loss of hope broke my heart. I am so grateful they were so supportive when I told them enough was enough and I wanted to walk into freedom again. They cheered me on and encouraged me every step of the way. I didn't have many friends at this stage of my life because my husband's job had us moving a lot. My network of encouragement was small, but it was mighty.

Do you have someone in your life who doesn't know the whole story, or doesn't even know a single part of it?

But what if you don't know who that might be? The first thing I would ask you to do is make a list of everyone in your life. People who are close to you, that is. Then identify the top two or three people you feel closest to and trust. You want to look for someone you truly trust won't tell anyone else and will absolutely be there for you, even if they don't understand. Ideally, you want to talk to someone who is a really great listener and not so much a "fixer." It's great to have someone come alongside you and encourage you, but speaking from experience, having someone just tell you exactly what they think you need to do is not the most helpful thing. It can be overwhelming and push you away from wanting to overcome your struggle!

Next you have to tell them. This is where you really get to choose the way that makes you most comfortable. I was pretty comfortable just talking it out with my husband, but this may not be the case for you. You could do it via email, a phone call, or even a handwritten letter if that feels a little less scary than a face-to-face conversation for you.

That's your homework: Go deep.

Don't worry, my recovering perfectionists, this homework won't be graded.

Strategy Three: Give Your Issues a Personality

We kind of touched on this when we talked about identity, but something I learned in counseling was to give your struggles a real name and personality. I did a long journaling exercise

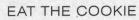

where I gave her these human characteristics, such as judgmental, shallow, and easily angered, then I asked her questions. For example, I asked her things like, "What do you want with me?" and, "Why did you leave me for so long and then come back?" And then, without overthinking, I just wrote the answers—whatever came to my mind first. You must go with your gut if you're going to do this, or you won't be able to get a clear picture. I felt like a fruitcake when I first did this exercise, but I promise that I found it *so* helpful. This was one of the ways I was able to identify my untrue thoughts and motivations for why I was doing what I was doing. When we identify those things, it allows us to figure out the opposite, feel the fear of what that is, but then do it anyway.

Strategy Four: Meet Jesus in Your Special Place

Meeting Jesus in my special place is another strategy I learned during my years of counseling and, yes, it may sound silly. But it works. Step one is identify this special place. This is any real place that has had great meaning to you in your life. For me, this was my childhood cabin. Sitting on the dock, overlooking the lake and feeling the sunshine dance across my skin was where I always felt the most happy and safe. This was my special place.

The next step is to tap into that big imagination I know you have and to imagine Jesus sitting next to you. It might take some time to get into this, and this kind of thing might not be for you, but once I began doing this, I felt this sense of peace—since Jesus is the Prince of Peace (Isaiah 9:6)—that allowed me to take a step out in faith, knowing he was right there on the dock with me. Whenever you feel yourself starting to build up that fear fortress, you can come back to this place, meet Jesus, and be able to continue to put one foot in front of the other.

Strategy Five: Look at Other Forms of Beauty

This strategy kind of blew my mind when I learned it from, you guessed it, counseling. I had never realized that the only body types I paid attention to were the ones I thought were "perfect." So I zoned in on girls I saw at the gym who had the body I wanted. Or I only paid attention to magazine covers that had fit, lean girls on them. I didn't see beauty in other bodies or, really, in any other thing. So I had to start paying attention to other forms of beauty. I started looking at other girls at the gym with bodies outside my idea of perfection and seeing how they could be beautiful. I saw the happiness on those girls' faces. I recognized that they have bodies that allow them to be healthy and move and breathe, and that is beautiful. I even looked at hairstyles and outfits of other women, because those things can be fun and beautiful too. I had to start finding beauty in other things and stop focusing only on what I thought would give me worth.

This might not apply to you if body image isn't your struggle, but it can still help to see beauty and wholeness in things other than whatever your image of perfection is. Maybe you look at someone who isn't a CEO and has more time to spend with friends. That kind of balance is beautiful. Maybe you look at a mom whose kids sometimes are a little crazy, and she doesn't always look put together. Instead of brushing her off and trying to find some other supermom to zone in on, you can pay attention. She shows up every day, she takes care of her kids, and she lets them be kids instead of trying to control them. That is a beautiful thing.

When we're able to see the meaning and beauty in things different from what we have told ourselves is the definition of beauty or perfection for so long, it makes it a whole lot less scary to take a step toward it ourselves.

And now, girlfriend, it's time to make your move.

FOR YOUR TOOLBOX

Peace I leave with you; my peace I give you. I do not give to you as the world gives. Do not let your hearts be troubled and do not be afraid.

—JOHN 14:27

I have told you these things, so that in me you may have peace. In this world you will have trouble. But take heart! I have overcome the world.

—JOHN 16:33

Let the peace of Christ rule in your hearts, since as members of one body you were called to peace. And be thankful.

—COLOSSIANS 3:15

And the peace of God, which transcends all understanding, will guard your hearts and your minds in Christ Jesus.

—PHILIPPIANS 4:7

DINNER RECIPE
MOROCCAN APRICOT CHICKEN

You don't have to wait for the weekend to get takeout from your favorite Middle Eastern restaurant. You can make it at home in only 20 minutes! This easy, weeknight chicken dinner is covered in a sticky, sweet, fruity apricot glaze with rich, flavorful notes of saffron that dance across your taste buds. A little smoky paprika, spicy cinnamon, and savory cumin balance out the sweetness in a way that makes this feel like a fancy restaurant dinner. My husband requests this one all the time!

Ingredients

For the glaze

1/4 cup apricot preserves

1/4 cup reduced-sodium chicken broth

1/8 teaspoon saffron (optional but recommended)

For the chicken

1 lb boneless, skinless chicken thighs (about 4 large thighs)

1 teaspoon cumin

1/2 teaspoon cinnamon

1/8 teaspoon smoked paprika

1/16 teaspoon allspice

Pinch of salt

1 tablespoon olive oil
cilantro for garnish

Directions

1. Combine the glaze ingredients in a small pot and bring to a boil on high heat. Once boiling, reduce the heat to medium-low and simmer until the glaze begins to thicken and reduce, about 3 minutes. Remove from heat and let stand to cool and thicken for 5 minutes.

2. While the glaze cools, cut any large chunks of fat off the chicken thighs and heat your oven to 400 degrees.

3. In a small bowl, stir together the cumin, cinnamon, paprika, allspice, and salt. Place the chicken in a large bowl and rub with the spice mixture until well coated.

4. Heat the oil in an oven-safe pan on high heat. Add in the chicken thighs and bake in the oven until the top is golden brown, about 2 minutes.

5. Flip the thighs and brush 2/3 of the glaze over them. Stick them back in the oven for 8–10 minutes, or until the thighs reach 165 degrees Fahrenheit.

6. Remove chicken from the oven and heat the oven to high broil. Brush the remaining glaze over the chicken and bake another 1–2 minutes.

7. Garnish with cilantro and serve!

PREP TIME: 5 minutes
COOK TIME: 15 minutes
SERVES: 4

TREADMILL TABATA WORKOUT

It's no secret that I am a lover of weights. But what many people don't know is that I do not love cardio. I'm not a runner, and I do not think I ever will be. I prefer to get my cardio through heavier weight circuits like the barbell complex.

However, I really enjoy getting my cardio through a Tabata workout. Tabata training was developed in Tokyo and is a timed interval method, kind of like high-intensity interval training. But the intervals are very short and very intense. A Tabata workout will alternate between 20-second intervals performed at your maximum effort, followed by 10 seconds of rest. You repeat this cycle 8 times and end up with an *awesome* workout that is only 4 minutes!

This kind of workout is ideal for busy schedules that don't allow a lot of time to get a workout in. While it is short, it is definitely not sweet. You will feel very tired and very sweaty after you complete a Tabata workout. But you will also feel totally energized and ready to take on your day!

Personally, I only do one day of true cardio a week because doing too much cardio can negatively impact sleep, hormone balance, recovery, and a whole bunch of other things. This

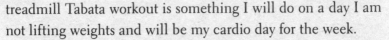

treadmill Tabata workout is something I will do on a day I am not lifting weights and will be my cardio day for the week.

To do this workout, start by running at an all-out sprint—whatever that means for you—for 20 seconds. Start slower and work your way up, listening to *your* body. Then quickly jump onto the rails of the treadmill (where the belt isn't moving) and rest for 10 seconds. Complete this workout for 8 intervals! Remember to drink your water on those rests!

Once you complete this, you'll be hooked on Tabata training. It's a great workout in a short time period—the best of both worlds!

The Workout

20 SECONDS ALL-OUT TREADMILL SPRINT

10 SECONDS RESTING ON THE SIDE RAILS

One set equals 1 round of sprints with 1 round of resting. Repeat until you have done 8 sets.

CHAPTER 8

THINK ABOUT WHAT IS TRUE AND LOVELY

You are my sunshine, my only sunshine.

—MY MOMMA (ALTHOUGH I'M PRETTY SURE THAT'S A REAL SONG NOT MADE UP BY HER)

ou're the devil!" I screamed at my doctor with fat, hot tears streaming down my face as my dad carried me over his shoulder out the door. She had just told me I was medically unstable and would need to be admitted to the hospital that evening. Thoughts started racing through my thirteen-year-old mind:

"She just wants to make you fat. She doesn't care at all about you."

"You're not medically ill. You're just skinny. You don't need help."

"They're going to make you ugly."

"Hmmm. How many calories did I eat for breakfast?"

I believed all these thoughts bouncing around my brain. I believed that the doctor did not want me to get healthy and had ulterior motives. These thoughts became seared into my brain, and I had no way to fight back. I sat in the back of my car, pinned to the seat in fear, as the thoughts kept coming. Frozen. Unable to make a move.

Growing up, I was probably one of the most optimistic and sunniest little kiddos you ever met. I always said I wished I could give my twin brother some of my "happy thoughts" when he was sad. I'm sure this is partly just genetics and partly that being a kid is a lot easier than being an adult, but I attribute some of it to my momma singing "You Are My Sunshine" to me almost every day. She told me I was sunshine, she told me I made her happy, and I believed that about myself. Because I had those positive thoughts and beliefs in my head, I was a happy kid.

But then I grew up.

It's not that my momma stopped singing this to me (she still does sometimes to this day), I just turned into this jaded teenager who didn't think Mom singing to her was awesome anymore. I also had started to live in the world, believing what the world was telling me about myself and what I needed to be or look like was true. Thoughts of becoming inadequate and worthless if I didn't look a certain way, have perfect relationships, or become successful in my career crept in. When I think way back to my early teen years, at the height of anorexia, my thoughts are really what started it all.

The thought of being more accepted if I was prettier.

The thought that getting prettier equated to being skinny.

The thought that getting skinny meant eating a lot less and moving a lot more.

The thought that if I gained weight, I would become worthless.

And so on.

Unfortunately, because history can repeat itself if we let our guard down, this all happened again in my early twenties.

The thought that I was out of control when that guy broke up with me.

The thought that I needed to get "perfect" to get back in control.

The thought that perfection could be attained with a perfect body.

And there's the Perfection Pursuit.

Girlfriend, what we focus on is what we believe. When I focused on being that sunshine, I *was* that sunshine. But when I focused on my goal of perfection, I did anything I needed to do to get there. I counted grapes, ate purse chicken, and even brought egg whites on first dates. I worked all day, ignored my husband, and barely slept. I believed I had to have the perfect body and make a lot of money to be worthy because those are the thoughts culture put in my brain.

Maybe you haven't had the exact same struggles, but I am willing to bet that your current struggles are coming from what you are focusing on and believe to be true. If you are focusing on your goal of workplace dominance, you probably believe your status gives you worth as a human because you'll be considered powerful and intelligent. If you're focusing on your goal of being a supermom, you probably believe your ability to parent is linked to your value as a woman, and so on and so on. But have you ever actually stopped to think about your beliefs and where they come from? Your thoughts are where *everything* starts.

Not only is what we think about what we believe, but those beliefs also become how we live our life. Don't get me wrong, I really enjoy eating food that makes me feel good and moving my body, but not to the extreme that I thought I did. I told myself that to be seen as special and worthy, I needed that perfect body. To get that perfect body, I needed to lift weights XYZ times each week and eat XYZ calories. Because I *thought* that was the math equation that equaled perfection, my actions led me down that dark and scary Perfection Pursuit. It started in my mind and then became actions in my life. And those thoughts took me so far away from God. I was so busy trying to figure out the perfection equation that I had no space in my brain left for God. When there is no space for someone, it's pretty hard to have a relationship with them.

The same thing can happen if you think being a supermom will give you worth as a woman. You may start acting like an annoying helicopter mom to make sure your kids are always behaving, since you believe their behavior reflects on you. If you believe being a CEO will bring you more worth because people will view you as a powerful woman, you may start missing out on the joys of life like getting together with friends, which could lead to isolation and burnout. There are many other examples I could give you, but it all comes down to this: We're always going to walk the walk that begins in our thoughts.

To get that thought life, and ourselves, back on track, we're going to have to start fighting a battle. Joyce Meyer says the mind is a battlefield,[1] and I agree 100 percent. No, I do not mean there are little army men running around shooting guns up there and that's why you get headaches sometimes, but there is a battle going on inside your pretty little head, and it's a battle for your thoughts.

Ephesians 6:12 says, "For our struggle is not against flesh and blood, but against the rulers, against the authorities, against the powers of this dark world and against the spiritual forces of evil in the heavenly realms." Girlfriend, there's a spiritual battle going on inside that head of yours. I used to believe I was the person thinking all these thoughts, so I was basically fighting a battle against myself. Can I just be real with you? When you think you're waging a war against yourself, it's a lose-lose situation. When you win, you still lose. And when you lose, you still lose. I know, it sounds totally confusing, but if you sit and think about it, it makes sense.

But this battle is not against ourselves. It's a battle against the spiritual forces of evil in the heavenly realms. I'm willing to bet you already know who that is. If you said the enemy, you are correct! He's prowling around your brain using that lie of "Did God really say?" over and over. Beginning to doubt who we are and what God says starts in the mind, so that is where the enemy attacks. I doubted what God said about my being fearfully and wonderfully made (Psalm 139:14) was true, so I tried to take matters into my own hands. If the enemy had not planted those seeds of doubt in my brain, I would never

171

have put one foot in front of the other and walked down the Perfection Pursuit.

Truth be told, I was so busy focusing on the thoughts of doubt, insecurity, and fear the enemy had rooted into my brain that I didn't even think about God, let alone what he said about me. There was zero space in my thought life for God when I was on the Perfection Pursuit. I can't tell you how many devotionals I had on my table collecting dust because I just didn't have time for a relationship with God.

Another goal of the enemy is to get you so wrapped up in your own brain that you don't have time to look up. He wants you to look out and identify the areas of culture that will give you worth, and then he wants you to look inside yourself to see how you can achieve that. He wants to keep you nice and busy. He wants you to be running around like a ridiculously annoying hamster in a wheel, feeling like you're chasing something worthy, but in reality, you're just going nowhere really, really fast.

The enemy doesn't want you to think about what God says about you. He doesn't want you to think about God at all. He loves to have you wrapped around his ugly little finger, thinking untrue thoughts and acting them out in your life. He loves when you head down that dark and scary Perfection Pursuit that leads you to misplaced worth and value. Heck, he probably even laughs when we trip and fall right into the biggest, stickiest, nastiest cobweb.

Another tool the enemy uses to keep our brains way too full to think about God is overthinking. Man. Oh. Man. Overthinking is something so many of us struggle with. Overthinking can be similar to future tripping, where we start thinking about all the things that *could* go wrong in a situation, or we decide in advance that something will turn out badly, so we don't take any kind of action forward. Our thoughts can motivate our actions, but overthinking will almost always cause inaction. The enemy doesn't always cause us to think about things that lead our actions down the wrong path, but sometimes he causes us to overthink ourselves into frozen statues. Not moving. Scared to take the next step, and definitely scared to take a step out in faith toward God. Overthinking caused me to question my doctor and believe she did not have my best interests in mind. It caused me to feel like I had no power.

I thought myself into taking the steps to achieve what I thought would give me an identity, and then I overthought myself into staying there. We don't usually realize we've thought ourselves down the wrong path until we're deep in the woods. At that point, we're primed and ready to overthink about all the things that could go wrong if we turn around, because isn't walking back that way what we were walking away from in the first place? And so, we're stuck.

Girlfriend, did you know you can think about what you're thinking about? I know that sounds totally strange, but *think* about it. I used to think my thoughts were just out of my control. When I thought a thought, I didn't even question if it was true. I didn't even question why it was just hangin' out in my brain. I would get so wrapped up in thinking about what I was going to eat later, what I had already eaten, when I was going to eat, and how many calories I had eaten *every single day*. Because these thoughts were always there, I just assumed I had to think about them until they finally left.

Is this you too? Are you overthinking everything? Maybe you are overthinking what you need to do to be the best mom when, really, your kids just need you to show up and support them. Or you are overthinking how to have the perfect relationship when it's truly just about loving, trusting, and supporting the other person. Are you just thinking all the thoughts that pop into your brain without even asking yourself why they are there? Well, I have good news for you!

Second Corinthians 10:5 says we can take our thoughts captive and make them obedient to Christ. Remember, there is a battle for your mind going on, so we're using strong words like "captive." This isn't sunshine and unicorns. You can't just put your thoughts in a box under your bed and hope they will leave you alone. This is a *war*, and you are a *warrior woman*, so take those thoughts captive!

My definition of a captive is someone who is being held back from living their best life by someone or something that doesn't have their best interests in mind—someone who has been taken prisoner. If you've done some of the exercises in this book, you've already given your negative thoughts a name and a persona. If you haven't, use your imagination and pretend your thoughts are a person. What happens when people are taken prisoner? They are usually confined to a room and questioned about where they came from and who sent them. So we have to do the same things to our thoughts. We must zone in on them, separate them from all our other thoughts, and then question and test them.

We don't need to ask who sent them because any negative thought always comes from the enemy. Psalm 149:4 says the Lord delights in us, and Genesis 1:27 says he made us in his image, so he would never fill our heads with negative thoughts about ourselves. God would not be putting himself down. Even though we know where these thoughts come from, we still have to take them captive and compare them to what Scripture says and expose them for the lies they are.

We can start by asking if our thoughts line up with Philippians 4:8: "Whatever is true, whatever is noble, whatever is right, whatever is pure, whatever is lovely, whatever is admirable—if anything is excellent or praiseworthy—think about such things."

Thinking, "I'm fat" is definitely not lovely.

Thinking, "I'm the worst mom on the planet" isn't admirable.

Thinking, "I will never measure up to that person on social media" isn't right or true.

Thinking, "If I were prettier, I could be more valuable" isn't pure.

Thinking, "I'll sacrifice all my social life (and maybe even my time with God!) to get that promotion" is definitely not noble.

These are the questions we can ask our thoughts. Are they true, noble, right, pure, lovely, or admirable? When I started my hospital recovery, I learned about this Bible verse and learned I was able to question my thoughts like this. I soon realized that the thoughts I had about the doctor and her motives were not true and that I could fight back against untruth. I didn't have to stay frozen and powerless to those thoughts. Questioning our thoughts is the first step toward identifying if a thought is worth thinking about, or if we should tell it to hit the road.

When you first start to do this, it might be a little bit challenging. We are used to letting these thoughts roll around our brains all day long without even realizing it. It's just a natural thing that happens, which makes it really hard to stop. You're going to have to be very intentional in thinking about what you're thinking about. This was so hard for me. I could start eating more and moving less, but taking these thoughts captive and making them obedient to Christ was *not* easy. Knowing I *could* do this but not *being able* to do it was one of the most frustrating experiences in my walk with God.

But you know that annoying saying "Practice makes perfect"? It's *true*.

When I truly started to be intentional about assessing the thoughts that were hanging out in my brain and turning into the very actions I was taking, it became a lot easier. Soon I found myself wandering around the grocery store looking at fun new foods to buy. I'd stumble across something delicious but not "clean," and I would want to buy it *so* bad, but those ugly thoughts would pop up and say, "Um, no. That is going to make you fat." Before I realized that I could think about what I was thinking about, I would put the jar down and walk away with some low-fat sad peanut butter that would probably take me two years to eat because I could only have one tablespoon per day.

PSA: A life where you can eat only one tablespoon of low-fat peanut butter per day is *not* a life you want to be a part of.

But eventually I started to fight back and ask questions like, "How is that true? Matthew 6:25 tells me not to worry about my body, or what I will eat or drink."

And then, *silence*.

Of course, those thoughts would come right back again pretty soon. But the voice became a whisper, and those whispers became few and far between. I was able to stop feeling frustrated with God and slowly start to give those thoughts over to him.

I am not going to lie to you and say those thoughts never come around anymore. There are days when it takes me a little longer than I'd like to admit to take those thoughts captive, but because I've been practicing, those days are fewer and fewer.

You may be thinking, "That sounds really awesome, Taylor, but once I identify a thought that isn't true, how do I fight those lies with truth when I don't even know what the truth is?" This is where you get to play detective and start finding Scripture that speaks to your soul. If you don't do a little digging around the Bible, you won't be ready to take your thoughts captive and fight back.

When I was sitting in that hospital bed, I started a Scripture journal. I gathered a ton of verses that spoke to me—verses on fear, verses on being made in God's image, etc.—and wrote them down. Every week I would memorize one verse. The next week, I would repeat last week's verse every day, and then move on to the new verse for the week. I now have about thirty verses memorized and still cycle through them once every morning to keep them fresh. Then I can use them as my battle swords throughout the day when I need them. I also keep the journal close by so I can add verses as I find them. I'm not saying you *need* to do this, but it's something that has really helped me.

When we start to identify our thoughts, and we start measuring them against what God says, we can begin to take back our thought lives. Taking back our thought lives will lead to taking back our whole lives, pointing us up to God, and allowing us to experience the fullness of his joy and freedom.

Because I like you, I've already done a little digging for you to get you started on your own Scripture journal!

LIE: I am not enough.

TRUTH: You are chosen by God, his special possession. He called you out of darkness into his light (1 Peter 2:9).

LIE: I am not beautiful.

TRUTH: Your beauty doesn't come from the outside. It comes from a gentle and quiet spirit. *This is what is worthy to God* (1 Peter 3:3–4). Also, you are fearfully and wonderfully made (Psalm 139:14)!

LIE: I can't do this. I'm a failure.

TRUTH: God is always there to help and strengthen you. He is holding you up (Isaiah 41:10).

LIE: If I could just have XYZ, then I would be happy.

TRUTH: God will supply everything you *truly* need (Philippians 4:19). Also, God will fill you with joy, peace, and hope as you trust in him, not in the things of the world (Romans 15:13).

LIE: I'm too far gone. I can't turn back to who I was and want to be.

TRUTH: When you are in Christ, you are a *new creation*! Seek him now, and all the old stuff will become new (2 Corinthians 5:17).

I once heard author and speaker Nicole Unice say our anxiety and fear can give us a picture of what a moment-by-moment relationship with God looks like.[2] We are constantly bombarded with these anxious, fearful thoughts *all day long.* Can you imagine what our life would be like if every time we experienced these thoughts, we went to the Lord? If every fearful thought triggered us to spend time with him, that would be one heck of a serious relationship with God. This is something I am currently trying to practice, and my relationship with God is deeper than it ever has been.

The first step to this kind of relationship with God would be to take that fear thought captive and go to the Scripture journal I know you're going to read when things get a little crazy up in your head. Or you might already have your favorite verses memorized, so you can just start repeating them over and over in your brain, stabbing your Scripture sword into that untrue thought with every verse you repeat.

Once you've begun to take your thought life captive, you may just want to put on your scuba suit and go a little deeper. When those fear thoughts come around (and they always will), you can turn them into a real relationship builder with God that goes beyond just repeating Scripture in your head by adding prayer and spending more time with him, uncovering more of his truth, and adding what you learn to your arsenal of truth bombs to blow up the enemy.

That, girlfriend, is a moment-by-moment relationship with God, not just one where you spend twenty minutes doing a devotional in the morning while not really focusing because you're thinking about all the other things you must do that day. When you're able to turn to God, knowing his truth and fighting on the battlefield for your mind, moment by moment, in real life, *that* is when you get serious. And that is when you get *seriously* free.

If you've read any part of this book, you already know I love sharing my nuggets of knowledge gained from the many years I've spent sitting on couches babbling to strangers about my purse-chicken, grape-counting ways. So, you guessed it, I have some helpful tactics for taking back your thoughts.

One of the simplest and most effective tricks for me was the "stop-sign trick." When a nasty little thought starts hanging out in your brain, close your eyes and imagine a stop sign. This works for a few reasons. First, when you're working *really* hard to use your imagination, your brain cannot be thinking about something else. You're taking up way too much brainpower to do any other kind of thinking. So you nipped that little thought right in the bud.

It also works because, after some time, your brain will start associating the fear thoughts that pop into your mind over and over with this stop-sign image. As humans, we already know what to do when we see a stop sign in real life, so this also starts to happen with fear in your brain. Think of your brain as a Ferrari driving down your thought highway. When it comes across a nasty thought, a big stop sign pops up, and eventually you'll stop thinking about it. Over time, those thoughts will be fewer and farther between.

This stop-sign trick, in conjunction with taking my thoughts captive and aligning them with Scripture, has been powerful for me.

The second trick is to not give in to the tantrum of your thoughts. You know when you see a kid at the grocery store having a temper tantrum because he wants a cookie? Then the poor, frazzled momma who just wants to grocery shop in peace buys him one to calm him down? We all know that is just telling him that every time he gets all freaked out at the store, he's going to get a cookie. Your thoughts are kind of like small children having temper tantrums. Every time they appear in your head and you believe they are true and let them turn into real-life actions, you give in. You give that little boy a cookie. You know what that means, right? You're telling your thoughts that every time they come into your pretty little head, you will believe them, and you will do (or not do!) what they tell you because you believe them. But when you deny them, you're telling your thoughts that this is not okay and does not lead to them getting their way, and they leave.

You already know I'm going to say that not giving in to the tantrum means going to God's truth and fighting back with your truth-bomb arsenal. I don't need to tell you that again. You can also just start thinking the *opposite* of those unwanted thoughts. That's like giving the little boy a piece of broccoli instead of a cookie, and we all know that just would not fly.

When I started to try to change thoughts like "you're fat" to "dang girl, you're cute" or "if I don't work out today, then I'm a lazy, useless person" to "if I don't work out today it's because my body is tired, and normal people are tired," the tantrums started to stop.

Depending on your struggles, you can also physically *do* the opposite. For example, if you struggle with fear foods, like I did, you may have a lot of tantrums when those fear foods would come into play. Thanksgiving was a nightmare. And Christmas? Forget about it. When a cookie came around and my brain started doing its overthinking, future-tripping thing and went, "Oh heck no! Do not eat that one cookie because you will then be fat and unworthy," I would eat the cookie. This was effective in my work life too. If my brain told me to keep working all day or I would never ever get everything done and my whole business would explode, I would close my computer. Guess what? What the fear told me would happen didn't happen. When we do the opposite of the tantrum, the tantrum stops.

Now, if you struggle with food, actually *doing* the opposite thing will take you some time because, coming from personal experience, this is a *very* scary thing. I have been starting to take these steps only very recently. Start looking to Jesus, focus on those stop signs, and show that toddler in your brain who's in charge, and you'll start walking in freedom.

All our issues and struggles truly do start in our brains. What we focus on becomes our life. It becomes our belief system, and it will affect how we feel about ourselves, how we feel about others, the relationships we're in, and the actions we take throughout our day. But, girlfriend, you do not have to let them rule over your life for one more second.

You, my friend, are a *powerful* woman, and you have the power of Christ. You choose what to think about. Take that power back.

FOR YOUR TOOLBOX

Do not conform to the pattern of this world, but be transformed by the renewing of your mind. Then you will be able to test and approve what God's will is—his good, pleasing and perfect will.

—ROMANS 12:2

Set your minds on things above, not on earthly things. For you died, and your life is now hidden with Christ in God.

—COLOSSIANS 3:2–3

Search me, God, and know my heart;
    test me and know my anxious thoughts.
See if there is any offensive way in me,
    and lead me in the way everlasting.

—PSALM 139:23–24

"For my thoughts are not your thoughts,
    neither are your ways my ways,"
    declares the LORD.

—ISAIAH 55:8

DINNER RECIPE

MOROCCAN ROASTED CARROTS AND BEETS

Eating vegetables doesn't have to be bland and boring! These roasted beets and carrots are tossed with a spicy, Middle Eastern spice blend, roasted to crispy perfection, and are then tossed with creamy goat cheese, fresh herbs, and crunchy almonds. A drizzle of sticky-sweet honey balances out all the spiciness. My veggie-hating husband requests these vegetables on the regular.

Ingredients

1 tablespoon slivered almonds

6 medium rainbow carrots, sliced

4 small golden beets, sliced

1 tablespoon extra-virgin olive oil

$\frac{1}{2}$ teaspoon cinnamon

$\frac{1}{4}$ teaspoon cardamom

$\frac{1}{8}$ teaspoon allspice

Sea salt

2 tablespoons goat cheese, crumbled

3 tablespoons cilantro, minced

2 teaspoons fresh mint, minced

Dukkah seasoning

Honey

Directions

1. Preheat your oven to 400 degrees. Spread the almonds on a small pan and cook until golden brown—about 3–5 minutes. They burn quickly, so watch them closely!
2. Place the carrots and beets in a large bowl and toss with the olive oil.
3. In a separate, small bowl, mix together the cinnamon, cardamom, and allspice. Sprinkle over the vegetables and toss until evenly coated.

4. Spread the vegetables on a sheet pan in a single layer, leaving space between them, and sprinkle with salt. Bake until crispy and golden brown, about 15–20 minutes, stirring halfway through.
5. Once cooked, place the vegetables into a bowl and stir in the goat cheese, cilantro, mint, and a few shakes of Dukkah.
6. Divide between plates, drizzle with a little honey (about 1 teaspoon or so), and devour!

PREP TIME: 10 minutes
COOK TIME: 20 minutes
SERVES: 3–4 people, as a side

Pro Tips!

1. To ensure your vegetables get done at the same time, cut them roughly the same size.
2. Got an air fryer? This recipe works great that way too!
3. Make sure you leave some space between your vegetables when you roast them. If you don't, you will just steam them, and they won't get nice and crispy.
4. Dukkah is a Middle Eastern spice blend that can be found in the international aisle at many grocery stores or at specialty food stores.

FULL-BODY BLASTER 10-MINUTE KETTLEBELL WORKOUT

You don't need to spend hours at the gym to get a great workout! If you up your intensity, you really only need ten minutes. Kettlebells are an awesome way to get in a workout because they stimulate your muscles and give you a cardio workout at the same time. You can increase your strength and build up your speed and endurance all at the same time. Better yet, they take up very little space, so you can even do this workout at home!

This is a "ladder style" workout, so you're going to start with 10 reps of each exercise, followed immediately by 9 reps of each, immediately into 8, and so on until you're only doing 1 rep of each exercise. That is when you're done! This sounds simple and easy, but it is *tough*! So rest as much as you need to between sets, trying to get faster and rest less each time you do it.

If you want to be really crazy, you can do this at the end of a standard weight workout as a "finisher."

The Workout

LADDER (BEGINNING WITH 10 REPS EACH, 9, 8, 7 . . . 1)

BURPEES

KETTLEBELL SWINGS (USE ONE KETTLEBELL)

KETTLEBELL SQUAT AND PRESS[3]

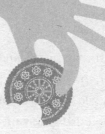

CHAPTER 9

EMBRACE
THE ALMOST
BUT NOT YET

Almost.
It's a big word for me.
I feel it everywhere.
Almost home.
Almost happy.
Almost changed.
Almost, but not quite.
Not yet.
Soon, maybe.
　　　　　　　—Joan Bauer

It was a wintery Saturday night, and my husband wanted to make pasta. That's right, handmade pasta because we're ambitious like that. He wanted to open a bottle of that wine he knows I like, put on some Spanish guitar music, and have a romantic date-night in. I've watched quite a few romantic movies in my life, and this date-night sounded like something from one of those. Of course, I said yes. We went to the grocery store to browse around and see what ingredients looked good for some stuffed pasta. I went into the store feeling excited about this ultra-romantic night we were going to have. I mean, Spanish guitar music, pasta, and wine? I am here for it. I had come so far in my journey with walking away from the Perfection Pursuit, and it felt like this would be a celebration of where I was now. But as the hubs started to load fatty meats, cream, and even some *dessert* into the cart, the anxiety in me started to bubble up.

We got home and the Spanish music came on. The wine was poured. We began the pasta making. Anxiety was rising higher and higher. How many calories were in that pasta? How was I going to eat carbs *and* drink wine at the same time? "Focus, Taylor. Focus on your husband. Focus on romance." Stop sign goes up. Matthew 6:25 tells me not to worry about what I will eat or drink. Okay, feeling better.

"Oh man, now it's time to eat the pasta. I don't know how to do this. This is hard. Why am I still so focused on the pasta and not on the person I am making it with, or the time we are spending together? Why can't I just be free of my food obsession? Why am I so darn stuck? I came into this date-night *so* excited, so ready to do something fun and romantic, and now here I am, right back where I started."

Girlfriend, this is a real-life peek into my thoughts from a date-night not so long ago, a night when I had been actively pursuing freedom, thinking about true and lovely things, digging deep into where my obsessions and fears were coming from, and feeling the fear and doing things anyway. I had been taking huge steps, but I found myself stuck.

If you're wondering, I did eat the pasta and drink the wine. Only to go to bed, cry my eyes out, and get into an argument with my husband because I took my anxiety and fears out on him.

We've learned there is no such thing as perfection, and the Perfection Pursuit will always leave us feeling unsatisfied. We've figured out our worth, and where it's been misplaced. We've identified our need for control, our deep fears, and the fig leaves we use to cover up our shame. Heck, we even started taking back our thoughts and stickin' it to Satan with memorized Scriptures. We're throwing those stop signs up left, right, and center, and feeling the fear but *doing it anyway.* We are kickin' butt and takin' names in the fight to reclaim our true identities and walk into the freedom God has for us.

We are making progress. We are taking steps. We are starting to taste freedom.

That, my friend, is exactly where the enemy does *not* want you to be. The enemy knows that when you come to Christ, he is left over on the losing side.

So why do we suddenly feel stuck?

How can we believe we are altogether beautiful and flawless (Song of Solomon 4:7) if the world says we aren't beautiful unless we have a thigh gap? How can we believe we are chosen by God (1 Peter 2:9) if the man we like doesn't choose us?

And how can we believe we are made brand-new in Christ (2 Corinthians 5:17) if we feel broken and shattered inside?

This is where I spent years, and I bet this is where you may have found, or still find, yourself as well. I felt like I was doing all the "right" things to walk with God, and I was so ready in my head for full freedom. Yet I wasn't able to fully trust God and step out in full surrender. It felt like ramming up against a wall over and over again, almost about to jump up and scale it. But every time I got close to getting over it, the enemy would push me right back down.

I remember a sermon in church about how many of us live out our lives with one hand behind our backs. We tell God we are in full surrender to him, but there is something we are too scared to part with. It's like we hold it behind our backs thinking that if we act like we are giving it up to him, God won't be able to see it. We're all adults here and know that your average human can see when you have a hand behind your back, so why do we feel like God, the maker of the universe, can't?

I would face my food fear and go out for big, bad, scary pizza Saturday night, only to go to church the next day and start singing a song about being free in God. I was singing the song with my mouth, but not at all with my heart. My heart and head were still focused on the Saturday-night pizza situation and what it would do to my body. I'd spend the rest of the worship in tears, wondering why I didn't have freedom even though I was taking all these steps.

Seriously, at some point I should have just learned my lesson and stopped wearing mascara to church.

When we're trying to break free from the Perfection

Pursuit, redefine our identities, and break down the walls of our fear fortresses, that freedom we so crave can turn into an idol. I know you and I are good-intentioned kinds of people, so we don't mean for this to happen, it just kind of naturally does. When we have been living one way for so long and then try to do a complete 180, it takes some time for the new way of life to really sink in, and so our natural inclination is to still look for something to give us meaning and value. I told myself I wanted to give up my food and body-image idolatry right here, right now, and I was ready to do it.

Then, when it didn't happen overnight, it wrecked me. I began to wonder over and over why I was constantly ramming up against a wall. Why was I not free? It wasn't until my counselor called me out that I realized it. She was the one that put the idea into my head that maybe I had turned from idolizing my body to idolizing my freedom. You know that feeling you have when you have some time off and you don't know what day it is, what time it is, or even if you're wearing pants? That's how I felt. I was just hit by this wave of confusion. How could all this striving for freedom end up in bondage to something else?

I stayed right there for a very long time. Years. Every morning feeling like today was going to be the day, only to end up eating my pre-measured grapes and some boring, undressed salad for dinner, crying to my husband that *I just wanted to be free.* Crying out to God too. Wondering why he wasn't just *giving it to me already*! When freedom became my everything, my life felt like bondage. Now, not only did almost all my thoughts revolve around food, calories, and body image, but whatever room I had left in my brain also revolved around wishing so

191

badly that those thoughts about food, calories, and body image would leave.

Sometimes they did. The stop-sign tricks, the Bible verses, and all the other tricks would work. Then some lies would slip in, and I'd feel like I wasn't free. I'd go back to obsessing about trying to return to the freedom I experienced for that short time. It was like this boxing match in my mind. In *this* corner: the idol of food! In *this* corner: the idol of freedom! Really, no one won that boxing match. It was always a tie. My life was riddled with false gods.

Maybe you can identify with this. You've figured out where you've misplaced your worth and value, are coming around to the idea of not being the perfect supermom, businesswoman, or college student, and you're starting to open your Bible to become a "good Christian girl" who has her Scriptures ready. You're doing it. I see you. I see you *trying*. I see you seeking out that cozy blanket of God's love, piling your hot chocolate with marshmallows, and trying to rest in that love and let it define you. If you're anything like me, you've read verses like Matthew 10:1, and you see the disciples casting out demons and healing people, and you're wondering why you don't have access to that kind of power. You have your stop signs ready, but you just can't stop the battle going on in your mind. You are headed down the Perfection Pursuit and thinking that wearing clothes made of fig leaves is totally high fashion right now. Freedom sounds so amazing, and you're fixating on it, but how does it actually, *truly* happen?

During these years, my walk with God wasn't the brightest nail polish in the box. It was more like that pretty color you use a lot at first, but then you get tired of it, so you throw it into the back of your makeup drawer where things go to die. When I first decided I was going to be free, and be free *now*, I was not really seeking out God. I believed all the Scriptures I had written down and memorized to counteract the lies, but freedom didn't come. I began to feel like David in Psalm 69, crying out to God to rescue me from the mire of my own life.

Luke 11:11 says, "Which of you fathers, if your son asks for a fish, will give him a snake instead?" I think, sometimes, when we start to do the hard work on ourselves and we begin to really seek God and ask for his freedom and it doesn't happen, we think he is giving us a snake. This is how I felt, and I'm pretty darn sure you have felt this too. We have our poles in the water, waiting for that freedom fish to bite, only to get bitten in the booty by a snake. We can't treat God like a genie. We can't just rub our little magic lamp (in this case, that's prayer) and expect him to grant our wishes as soon as we want them and in the way that we want him to. It wasn't until I realized I was treating God this way that I understood that God wasn't giving me snakes, he was just giving me some seriously disguised fish. But, hey, disguised or not, a fish is sure better than a snake.

When my counselor called me out that day and made me realize I had been doing some idol hopping and transferring my body idolatry to a freedom idolatry, it made me realize God hadn't granted the cry of my heart for a reason. Psalm 37:4 says, "Take delight in the LORD, and he will give you the desires of your heart." My desire was freedom, but I wasn't delighting in the Lord, and that's why he wasn't giving me freedom—he wanted me to delight in him *first*. Which is pretty ironic because I had this verse tattooed to my rib cage long before I started wandering back down the Perfection Pursuit.

In hindsight, I never called to God and told him I just wanted him, that I wanted to be truly and wholly satisfied in him. I only cried out to him for what he could give me. In Natalie Grant's song "More Than Anything," she says, "help me want the savior more than the saving," and I wanted the saving more than the savior.

I also realized I was using control in my recovery from being a control freak! How backward is that? I would get my husband to weigh me on the scale to make sure I was gaining weight but giving up control of having to see that increase. Then I would bug him all day long to tell me how much I had gained. I'd ask him in the morning. I'd text him about it. I'd even ask him over the dinner table when I thought he would just be so annoyed and want to eat in peace that he would tell me. Sometimes I would even consider breaking into his phone, where he recorded my weight, when he wouldn't tell me. Don't look at me like that, I know you've done some lackluster things yourself. When we take a step toward freedom, sometimes we take a step that was just a *little* too big, and we have to backpedal. We go back to even controlling how we get to that freedom.

It always comes back to a misplaced freedom focus.

Deep down inside I was still relying on myself and my own methods to bring me the freedom I desired, without letting those actions come from a place of full surrender to God. Using mental stop signs, having tons of memory verses written down, and using them when the enemy is fighting for our minds are all great ways to fight the lies, but they only go so far. When you're just using the tools without allowing them to sink into your soul, they lose their power. When you're using them and expecting that the very act of using them is going to bring you to freedom, they lose their power.

No matter how many Bible verses we memorize, we are still humans. We will always fall short. I came to realize I had just been going through the motions. I did the things my counselor told me to do. Yes, they definitely helped a lot, but not to the point of total surrender that leads to freedom. I learned a ton of Bible verses and tried to always remember to go to them. Nope, still not free.

Then, one day I read James 1:23–25, which says, "Anyone who listens to the word but does not do what it says is like someone who looks at his face in the mirror and, after looking at himself, goes away and immediately forgets what he looks like. But whoever looks intently into the perfect law that gives freedom, and continues in it—not forgetting what they have heard, but doing it—they will be blessed in what they do." When I read that, it hit hard. Each and every day I had gotten up and told myself that today was the day, but every day I went on my way and totally forgot that conversation with myself, which is exactly like forgetting what you look like! I realized I wasn't actually *doing* the Word of God. I was just using tips and tricks to try to get better at using it for my own goals. But, girlfriend, we all know actions speak louder than words.

The second part of that verse brings so much hope—hope that if we actually go out and *do* the Word of God, without forgetting it, we will be blessed in what we do, and we will be given the freedom we so deeply yearn for.

I had to ask myself a hard question: Why am I forgetting

this every day? Why are all the good tips and tricks I've already shared with you not working? When I was really honest with myself, I came to the conclusion that although I truly believed *in* God, I did not believe *him*. I believed he created me. I believed he created you. I believed he created the world and he is all-powerful, all-knowing, and generally pretty awesome. But deep down I didn't truly believe that what he had was better for me or that he was truly in control. I didn't truly believe the joy of the Lord would be my strength (Nehemiah 8:10).

The things I have been teaching you are great, and they work, but not when you don't actually believe they will work and surrender completely to God. They will still have power when you use them, but if not backed up by true belief, they won't have the power you want them to have. After Googling "What does the Bible say about believing God?" I came across Numbers 23:19. It says, "God is not human, that he should lie, not a human being, that he should change his mind. Does he speak and then not act? Does he promise and not fulfill?"

The reason we tend to believe *in* God but not believe *him* is because we put our human experiences on God. We know people lie. We know people don't always have our backs, and so we can sometimes assume the same thing of God, even if we don't realize we have these assumptions. I know I was so guilty of this and, honestly, I still am at times. This verse in Numbers assures us otherwise, though. It assures us that God is *not* a human. He won't lie like a human. He won't change his mind like a human. And he won't promise us something and not fulfill it. He *does* have our backs, and we need to just allow ourselves to take our human experience out of the picture and be held in God's very capable hands, believing him *and* believing in him. Easier said than done, I know. But the more you trust him, the easier it becomes.

Another thing that can get in the way of believing God instead of just believing *in* him is pride. Does that word make you squirm like it makes me squirm? No one wants to think they are prideful, but we all are to some degree. When we don't believe God, it's because we think we have everything planned out much better than he does. In Proverbs 8:13, God says he hates pride and arrogance, and I assume it is because pride makes us look to our own strength and abilities instead of looking to the giver of those strengths and abilities. When we are focusing on ourselves, our pride gets in the way of even seeing God.

Look at the wall in front of you right now. For the purposes of this exercise, that wall is God. Now, take your hand and put it directly in your line of vision, between your face and the wall. Your hand is pride. You can't see the wall, right? You can't see God when pride is blocking your view. It's pretty hard to trust and believe in something and surrender your whole life to it when you can't even see it. Pride can be one of our biggest obstacles to glorifying God and achieving full freedom, and I know this is a struggle. I believed I truly knew what my body needed better than it did. I believed my brain more than the signals my body (the body God made) gave me. I also believed I could plan my future and my success. I didn't trust God in all those things, and so I couldn't see him clearly.

In Beth Moore's devotional *Breaking Free*, she says, "God's hatred of pride doesn't mean that he wants you to feel bad about yourself . . . God hates pride because it dethrones Him and puts ourselves at the center of the universe." She says, "God's hatred of pride expresses his love."[1] This is because he knows that when we are at the center, it only leads to our downfall.

When I finally realized I was doing all these good actions out of my *own* strength, and out of pride, I realized God was actually giving me a fish. He was teaching me that although all my actions were helping to win the battle in my mind, ultimately I already had everything I needed in him, and I needed to get out of my own way and truly believe him.

Girlfriend, isn't that *freeing* to read?

We know our citizenship is in heaven (Philippians 3:20), and we will eventually live in full freedom with God. But we live in this world right now, so we can't fully experience that. There is this tension of "almost but not yet" that leaves us wanting full freedom and joy in this life while realizing we will get it only when we live with God. Colossians 3:5 says, "Put to death, therefore, whatever belongs to your earthly nature," and part of the act of putting that nature to death is realizing we are free in this life, even when we struggle, because the battle has already been won.

Life is a constant journey, and we will always struggle to some degree, and that's okay. Realizing *that* is freeing. When we try to make freedom fit into our perfect box—what it should look like and how it should happen—that is when we feel stuck. I know you and I have been on the quest for perfection, but we have to be careful not to have our desire for finding freedom in God mask that we are still walking the Perfection Pursuit, or we will run into trouble. Our imperfection *is* our perfection, and there isn't a set finish line.

Maybe you will find full and total freedom in this life, and maybe you won't. But I can tell you that utilizing some of the tips and tricks I've shared and coupling them with truly learning to find your satisfaction in knowing Christ is enough is going to bring you closer and closer to freedom. Learning from our mistakes will always make us stronger. Remember, the battle is already won, and it's okay to feel the tension between where you are and where you want to be. The Perfection Pursuit is always waiting for us. But if we commit our lives to pursuing Jesus, we will find a joy that never ends. Just give yourself a little grace to be both a work in progress and a masterpiece at the same time.

FOR YOUR TOOLBOX

Since, then, you have been raised with Christ, set your hearts on things above, where Christ is, seated at the right hand of God. Set your minds on things above, not on earthly things. For you died, and your life is now hidden with Christ in God. When Christ, who is your life, appears, then you also will appear with him in glory.

—Colossians 3:1–4

For if you live according to the flesh, you will die; but if by the Spirit you put to death the misdeeds of the body, you will live.

—Romans 8:13

The world and its desires pass away, but whoever does the will of God lives forever.

—1 John 2:17

DESSERT RECIPE

TURMERIC GINGER CHOCOLATE CHIP COOKIES

The classic chocolate chip cookie, anti-inflammatory style! These chocolate chip cookies are the perfect combination of crispy on the outside and so soft and chewy on the inside. You will not believe they are gluten-free, dairy-free, and even egg-free. They get their bright yellow color and spicy-sweet taste from ginger and turmeric, which help digestion and fight inflammation. These pillowy-soft cookies are studded with ooey-gooey, melty chocolate chips in every bite!

Ingredients

1 1/2 cups oat flour (163g)

1 teaspoon cornstarch

3/4 teaspoon baking soda

1/2 teaspoon ground ginger

1/2 teaspoon turmeric

1/4 teaspoon salt

1/4 cup coconut oil, melted

6 tablespoons raw organic cane sugar

3 tablespoons coconut sugar

2 tablespoons water

1 tablespoon avocado oil

2 teaspoons baking powder
⅓ cup dark chocolate dairy-free chocolate chips

Directions

1. In a medium bowl, stir together the oat flour, cornstarch, baking soda, ginger, turmeric, and salt.
2. In a large bowl, beat the coconut oil and sugars together with an electric hand mixer until just combined.
3. In a separate small bowl, whisk together the water, avocado oil, and baking powder. Pour this mixture into the coconut oil mixture and beat on high speed until it begins to thicken, about 1 minute.
4. Add in the dry ingredients and stir until combined. Stir in the chocolate chips.
5. Cover and refrigerate until the dough just begins to firm up, about 20–30 minutes.
6. Once chilled, preheat your oven to 325 degrees and line a cookie sheet with parchment paper.
7. Scoop out a slightly heaping 1 tablespoon of dough. Roll into a ball and place on the prepared cookie sheet. Repeat with remaining dough. Press the balls down lightly—you want them higher than they are wide.
8. Bake until the tops feel *just* set (the rest of the

cookie will look quite soft), about 14–16 minutes. Let cool on the pan for 5 minutes.

9. Transfer to a wire rack to cool completely.
10. Devour!

PREP TIME: 40 minutes
COOK TIME: 15 minutes
YIELD: 14 cookies

Pro Tips!

1. Don't have oat flour? Put rolled, old-fashioned oats in a high-powered blender and blend for about 1 minute until powdery.
2. Don't like turmeric or ginger? Feel free to omit them for a standard chocolate chip cookie.
3. Don't have coconut sugar? Use brown sugar.

LIVING ROOM HIIT WORKOUT

I'm sure you've heard of HIIT workouts. They're very popular, and for good reason! HIIT, which stands for "high-intensity interval training," speeds up your metabolic rate, causing your metabolism to be higher for up to 48 hours after you finish the workout. This means the burn is still going after you finish your session!

HIIT combines high intensity and intervals into a short but effective workout—much like the treadmill Tabata workout. However, you don't need a treadmill to perform this HIIT workout. In fact, you don't need any equipment at all! The focus is on using your body weight to get your heart rate up and making sure it stays there, so no need for any kind of fancy equipment!

This workout uses 5 different exercises and will take you 15 minutes. You will do each exercise for 30 seconds, and then rest for 30 seconds before moving on to the next exercise. You'll do the next exercise for 30 seconds, then a 30-second break, and continue until you're at the end. Once you've done all 5 exercises, just keep repeating until you've been doing this circuit for 15 minutes. If you're a total beginner to HIIT, you might want to start with only 10 minutes.

HIIT is high intensity, and I typically don't recommend doing it more than twice a week. You always want to give your body enough time to recover, and doing too much of HIIT (or too much of anything) can lead to overtraining.

So make some space in your living room and prepare to get a great workout!

The Workout

JUMPING JACKS FOR 30 SECONDS

30 SECONDS REST

ALTERNATING JUMPING LUNGES FOR 30 SECONDS

30 SECONDS REST

BUTT KICKS FOR 30 SECONDS

30 SECONDS REST

MOUNTAIN CLIMBERS FOR 30 SECONDS

30 SECONDS REST

SQUAT JUMPS FOR 30 SECONDS

30 SECONDS REST

CHAPTER 10

WALK THE WALK
INTO FREEDOM

Everything I thought would be a big
deal, and kept me from freedom,
was really not a big deal. In fact,
it was such a small deal that you
can't even consider it a deal at all.

—ME

In the last chapter I told you a story of what was supposed to
be a romantic date-night in with my hubs and how it ended in
tears. In fear. In not being able to be present and enjoy the date
because I couldn't break through the bondage of the control
food had over me. This chapter picks up on the very next day.

This day was my day for change.

I woke up, my eyes red and puffy from crying myself to sleep. Mind you, I wasn't crying over some life-altering thing like a death in the family. I was crying because I had eaten pasta and drunk wine at the same time—one of my irrational fears—and now I was riddled with anxiety, the kind of anxiety that doesn't go away after a nice, restful sleep. It was the kind of anxiety that kept me up most of the night. The kind of anxiety that made me ugly cry to my husband. The kind of anxiety that made me fight with my husband and put a strain on our relationship. The kind of anxiety that I had no place for in my life.

"Something has to change. I've been trying for almost a decade, and here I am crying over noodles with sauce and wine. A *drink*. These are *not* things to be afraid of. I am not talking about bears or snakes or spiders. This is *food*," I thought to myself. I got out of bed, looked in the mirror, and said, "God loves me, and I am beautiful. Whether I have abs or not. Whether I'm 'fitness-queen Taylor' or just 'normal-person Taylor.' I am going to choose to believe that."

I walked out of my bedroom and, for the first time in eight years, I didn't ignore my hunger and tell it to wait until later because it was "too early to eat."

I walked into the kitchen and made myself pancakes.

Girlfriend, you and I both know pancakes mean *serious* breakfast business.

We *can* learn to embrace the "almost but not yet" stages of our lives that many of us will find ourselves in when we start to utilize Scripture as a sword to fight the enemy, as well as some of the other tips and tricks I've shared. We can understand that sometimes we won't find full freedom in this life but still know the battle is already won, and it's okay to feel the tension between where we are and where we wish we were. However, if we make the choice to believe God and start to put actions behind that belief, we will find freedom.

And I did.

That morning I woke up and decided I had had enough. I have some straight talk for you: I got tired of my own crap, and sometimes that is what it takes. I was tired of my own excuses for why I was still where I was—so ready to be free, but just not quite there. I was tired of saying I believed everything to be true about what God says about me and who he is, using all kinds of techniques to put that truth in my life, but knowing deep inside that I didn't really believe it.

I was tired of my actions not reflecting my belief. Sure, some of them did, but the big actions didn't line up with what I said I believed. I still got up and immediately worked. Then I went to the gym, only to come back and work, work, work the day away. I was exhausted at the end of the day, and the last thing I wanted to do was spend time with Jesus. If I did do it, it was not meaningful, and it didn't reflect a desire for a relationship with him. I was still eating "safe foods" for the most part, just eating more of them. I didn't go out of my comfort zone and just eat a cookie, and that proved I didn't really believe God would love me even if that cookie changed my body. Which it wouldn't.

Eat that darn cookie. Make sure it has lots of chocolate chips.

Sometimes we just need to have a "rock-bottom" moment when our situation *truly* hits us and we realize that, although we are taking steps and we are slowly becoming free, we are holding ourselves back from full and total freedom. We have to come to the realization that a little bit of freedom or quasi-recovery isn't enough for us. We want it all, and we won't settle for less. C. S. Lewis once said, "We are half-hearted creatures, fooling about with drink and sex and ambition when infinite joy is offered to us, like an ignorant child who wants to go on making mud pies in a slum because he cannot imagine what is meant by the offer of a holiday at sea. We are far too easily pleased."[1] You and I can be those children making mud pies in a slum when we get stuck in quasi-freedom. We don't trust God when he calls us to something better, and we're too afraid to try, so we swing back and forth between the highs and lows and never just rest in him.

Until we decide enough is enough.

The question I get most on social media and in emails is "How do you recover from an eating disorder or disordered eating, and what does the recovery from that look like?" I think talking to someone who has gone through it and come out on the other side is comforting, so I want to go deeper into that true recovery and what it looked like for me. Even if you never struggled from disordered eating or an eating disorder, I still think full recovery looks the same for whatever bondage has mastery over your life. You may not experience all the same things I did, like regaining a period, gaining weight, and going through periods of extreme hunger, but many of the things I had to change in order to achieve freedom will still be the same.

1. I had to cut out the actions that led me down the Perfection Pursuit, even if they seemed like healthy

actions, and replace them with actions that drew me toward God.

2. I had to do virtually the opposite of everything I had been doing.

We all know that the definition of insanity is doing the same thing over and over and expecting a different result, right?

Do you hate the saying "Actions speak louder than words" as much as I do? It's probably the most overused cliché on this floating blue and green sphere we call the Earth, but that's probably because it's just so darn *true*. I lived in the in-between for nearly a decade because I was doing all the right things, but I wasn't truly believing in them deep down in my soul. A lot of this uncertainty boiled down to not believing God because I didn't have a relationship with him. That's step one right there—changing that. We need to develop a relationship with him, which means we need to get rid of whatever is getting in the way of us doing that. Remember that hand/wall analogy? We have to get rid of the hand.

I'm not talking about just getting rid of pride in your life (although that is very helpful!), I'm talking about completely getting rid of an action in your life that is causing you to walk down the Perfection Pursuit. Matthew 5:30 says, "And if your right hand causes you to stumble, cut it off and throw it away. It is better for you to lose one part of your body than for your whole body to go into hell." If something is causing us to stay in bondage, we have to cut it out of our lives. We can't just walk away from it, we have to *run* away from it. Sprint from it if you have the energy!

Exercise is a fantastic thing. It's something we should all

do to keep our bodies and minds healthy. But exercising like I was isn't healthy. Going to the gym was a huge snare for me, and it kept me walking on down that Perfection Pursuit for a long time. Not only did it keep me wrapped up in my body, I always liked to exercise first thing in the morning, so it was the first thing I thought about. It took me a long time to realize I couldn't even call what I was doing exercise anymore, because exercise should improve our health and fitness, and the way I was exercising was not improving my health. It was an addiction. It was causing me to see such a direct link between food and exercise that I could only eat if I had exercised. And worst of all, it took me away from thinking about God and spending time with him in the mornings like I knew I should.

I don't know what action is taking you away from God and keeps ushering you down the Perfection Pursuit, but if you're serious about breaking free, you need to identify it. It might be something as small as waking up and immediately spending your morning checking your emails, or maybe it's an addiction to reading parenting blogs or magazines that only leave you feeling like you'll never be a Pinterest-perfect mom, and you don't measure up.

We're going to cut it out.

I stopped working out. Entirely. I won't lie to you and say I did it immediately. The roaring lion still wanted to devour me and whispered lies in my head, like I could just cut out my once-a-week cardio session and that would be enough because it was still changing my actions. After a couple of weeks, I soon realized it wasn't enough, and my addiction to exercise was still the same. I had to totally go all in and cut it out entirely.

I stopped, and not just for a week. I stopped for almost a year.

Instead of getting up and going to the gym, I got up and did a Bible study. I had to prove to myself that what God said about me was true, and there was no way I was going to do that without spending time with him, developing a relationship with him, and having it be the first thing I did every day. Girlfriend, this was quite possibly the hardest thing I've ever done in my life.

It's so easy to justify the things we do, even when we know they hurt us. I told myself exercise was healthy. I did it for stress relief and any other excuse you can think of. Maybe you tell yourself that looking at those parenting blogs is your "me time" and it's a little bit of time away from the kids. Or maybe you tell yourself that checking those emails is the thing that keeps your business thriving. But is it? Or is it just keeping you locked up in your fear fortress, stuck in quasi-freedom?

Not only did I have to replace my exercise with something God-honoring, I had to start doing the opposite of things I had been doing that had kept me addicted to controlling what my body looked like. Quitting exercise and replacing it with some Jesus time was doing the opposite, but exercise wasn't the only thing keeping me in bondage. Food was. Rather, not eating it was.

So, I had to eat food. A lot of it.

It started with a breakfast of pancakes. Then, every time I started to obsessively think about food, I ate it instead of just thinking about how I *wished* I could eat it. I had to flip the switch and do the opposite of the thing that kept me in bondage, so I ate. I ate as soon as I got up. I ate every few hours. I ate a post-breakfast snack, and sometimes even another snack after that. Whenever I thought of how I shouldn't eat food, which was always at the beginning, I ate food.

Mr. FFF used to call me the "hungry monster" because many of my days were just spent wandering around the kitchen, opening cabinets, trying to find something to eat, and getting nothing done. Of course, at the time I did not like this nickname because eating all the time was scary and made me feel bad. Now I can look back at it and laugh at what I must have looked like.

If you're reading this and you're recovering from an eating disorder, disordered eating, or hypothalamic amenorrhea[2] (where you lose your period due to low body weight and/or too much exercise), I want to warn you about something to expect called "extreme hunger." This is something you will probably experience if you're recovering from this kind of bondage, because when we finally start to eat after not eating for so long, our body gets *really* excited. It wants to throw a huge party with enough food for a massive crowd, but it only wants *you* to eat it. This freaked me out at the start. I was always hungry, and I was always eating, and I thought it would never end. But it did. I can now eat normally and do not feel the desire to eat my entire kitchen every single day. But you do have to go through this and listen to your body and trust that you are doing nothing wrong. Your body needs that food.

I kept doing all the tips and tricks I've shared with you—stop signs, using verses in my thoughts, meeting Jesus in our place—but the difference was that this time I was putting my money where my mouth was. I was walking the walk, not just talking the talk. My actions were speaking louder than my words, and any other cliché you can think of. I found that, this time, when I did these things, they stuck. They actually started to have power. I didn't feel like I was just ramming up against a wall over and over again with no ability to scale it. It was like the wall suddenly had pegs on it, and one by one, I was slowly able to climb up those pegs and maneuver myself up and over that wall.

It was not easy. You may not experience a lot of things I did, depending on what kind of bondage you're trying to break free from, but when I was pursuing full freedom and eating all the time without exercise, I naturally gained weight. I knew in my head it was healthy and it was something I needed to do, but that feeling of letting "fitness-queen Taylor" down was *very* strong at this point. It was hard to see my body softer and with what I thought was "extra" weight. I thought I would gain weight forever and ever and ever, but I didn't. Eventually the weight gain stopped even though I was still eating a lot and not exercising at all. God designed our bodies to know where they are happy, and we can trust they will get there and stay there.

I'm going to apologize for this comparison before I even make it because it's a little intense, but it's something that resonated so much for me. Someone once told me that when you kill something, it screams before it dies, and that is what I found to be true. When I was truly working to kill "fitness-queen Taylor," she started to scream *really* loud. Every morning I didn't go to the gym, or every time I ate something scary or, really, ate anything more than what I thought was "acceptable," "fitness-queen Taylor" screamed at me in a way I did not even know was possible. The voice that wanted me to turn around and go back down that dark and scary Perfection Pursuit got so incredibly loud that I almost could not hear myself some days. Some days I had to read my Bible and eat my food with tears running down my face because the screaming was almost too much.

But, girlfriend, we don't come this far to only get this far.

It got harder before it got better, but it did get better. I can promise you that when you start spending quality time with God, and especially when that quality time is replacing the time you used to spend doing something that left you shackled in chains, it gets easier. When your actions finally show that you believe God, somehow your mind starts to understand that and comes onboard. When you start to fight back the lies with truth, it's almost like your brain surveys your real-life actions and says, "Okay, I see we are doing things that prove we really believe this, and they are not just empty words." And when you fight back, it sticks. But you have to prove to yourself that this is for real, and the only way to do that is to go through the hard part. To run, not walk, in the other direction, and start taking real and true actions that will lead you to freedom.

That ugly voice will want to start screaming again, but when you step into full freedom, you develop a magical ability to recognize when that voice starts whispering, and you can shush it right out of your life.

The woman writing this book is so different from the woman I've been telling you about in the previous nine chapters. I'm sitting on my couch right now with a plate of snacks beside me because you almost never find me without a snack anymore. I went on a spontaneous date-night out for dinner with my husband last night, had wine, and was totally present in the conversation. I didn't go to bed and cry. I didn't even go to bed and think about what I had eaten. I just went to bed and fell asleep.

I didn't wake up and think about what I was going to eat that day or when I was going to work out. I just got up, spent time with God, made breakfast, and moved on with my day. I have my period back, and my body is healthy and working. I no longer think about food and my body 24/7. In fact, I don't really think about my body at all except for when I see it in the mirror. I have other things that bring me so much more life and joy, and honestly, the things I thought would be a really big deal, like gaining weight, are really not any kind of deal at all. People don't even notice! What they do notice, though, is that I am so much happier and full of life.

At the time of writing this book, I'm still not going to the gym. I'm still enjoying my slow walks with my "Jesus tunes" outside and doing yoga a few times a week. Mentally, I know I am ready to go back to the gym and exercise in a way that feels joyful and not controlling, and my husband agrees I could. But my body has been under almost a decade of abuse, and I know it will take more than a year to undo that, so I am being cautious and waiting so I can fully heal.

My current approach to food is very intuitive; I listen to my body. Most of the time, I enjoy eating nourishing, well-balanced meals because they satisfy me and make me feel good while eating and after eating. But sometimes I have an intense desire for a cookie (or two), and instead of fighting it like I used to, I can eat the cookie and *move on*. I don't sit and stew over it anymore because food is really just food. It's not calories or macros or something to try to control. I don't view foods as "good" or "bad," "healthy" or "unhealthy." Food does not carry morality, and I would challenge you to look at how you view food. Do you see it with labels, or is all food just food to you? I now know that my body is smart enough to figure out what to do with the food I give it, even if I give it too much on some days. I honor and trust the body God designed for me.

Of course, there are still days when my thoughts start to go off track, and I might do things I used to do, like question why I am hungry or why I'm craving a cookie. But with my newfound food freedom I'm able to look at those thoughts logically and know they are just lies from the enemy. No matter what the roaring lion tells us, there is nothing better than having the joy of being free to live the life God has for you, and the joy of knowing that Christ is enough.

So eat the cookie. Taste the joy. Savor your freedom.

A few devotionals I love and find very helpful:

Redefined Study, by Well-Watered Women
Breaking Free, by Beth Moore
Me, Myself & Lies, by Jennifer Rothschild

Helpful podcasts:

Real Health Radio
Beauty in Christ
Redefining Wellness
The Unbreakable You

DESSERT RECIPE

GLUTEN-FREE AND DAIRY-FREE "BOY BROWNIES"

These are a remake of the boy brownies I talk about in chapter 1! The original recipe was made from a cake mix, so I reworked it to be homemade and gluten-, grain-, and dairy-free. These brownies are extremely dense and chewy, which is exactly how I like my brownies. They have a layer of almond milk caramel sauce and roasted, crunchy pecans with melty chocolate chips, and are finished off with a layer of chewy brownie bliss. They are a chocolate-lover's dream!

Ingredients

For the caramel
1/2 cup coconut sugar
1/4 cup unsweetened almond milk
4 teaspoons ghee
1/2 teaspoon vanilla

For the brownies
1/2 cup pecans
1 1/2 cups almond flour (150g)
1/4 cup cocoa powder
1/4 teaspoon baking soda
1/4 teaspoon salt
1 cup coconut sugar

3 tablespoons coconut oil, melted

1 large egg

1 egg yolk

1 teaspoon vanilla

½ cup dairy-free mini chocolate chips, divided

Directions

1. Preheat your oven to 350 degrees. Spread the pecans on a small baking sheet and bake until golden brown and toasted, about 10–12 minutes. Remove from the oven, roughly chop, and set aside.

2. In a small pot, combine all the caramel ingredients and bring to a boil. Once boiling, reduce the heat to medium-low and cook until the mixture darkens, thickens, and reduces by about half, about 10–12 minutes. Set aside to cool while you make the brownies.

3. In a medium bowl, stir together the almond flour, cocoa powder, baking soda, and salt.

4. In a large bowl, using an electric hand mixer, beat together the coconut sugar and coconut oil until the coconut sugar is just moistened. Add in the egg, egg yolk, and vanilla, and beat until well mixed.

5. Stir the almond flour mixture into the egg mixture and beat until just combined. Finally, stir in ¼ cup of the chocolate chips.

6. Line the bottom of an 8 × 8-inch pan with parchment paper and rub the sides with coconut oil. Spread 2/3 of the brownie mix on the bottom of the pan and bake for 10 minutes.

7. Once baked, sprinkle the remaining chocolate chips and the pecans over the brownies. Finally, pour the caramel evenly over the top and then spoon the remaining brownie batter over the caramel.

8. Bake until the top is crisp and a toothpick inserted in the center comes out clean (you'll still see some melted chocolate on the toothpick), about 25 minutes. Let cool on the counter for 5 minutes.

9. After 5 minutes, place a cooling pad in your refrigerator and place the brownies on it. Cool in the fridge for 45 minutes.

10. Remove from the fridge and finish cooling on the counter.

11. Slice and devour!

PREP TIME: 15 minutes
COOK TIME: 35 minutes
YIELD: 12 brownies

Pro Tips!

1. Always weigh your flour to ensure accurate results. Measuring cups can vary slightly, so

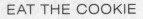

this is the easiest way to make sure these brownies turn out!

2. If you don't have ghee, you can use 5 teaspoons of butter. Ghee is a little richer than butter, so you need a little more of it to make up for the ghee.

3. I find it is easiest to use very lightly damp hands to spread the brownie mix into the pan and to crumble it on top of the pecans and chocolate chips.

4. Putting the brownies in the refrigerator cools them rapidly and makes them really chewy. But don't leave them in the refrigerator longer than 45 minutes or they will dry out.

DECK-OF-CARDS WORKOUT

Working out doesn't have to be grueling. It can be fun and keep you guessing, like this deck-of-cards workout! This one is fun because you can customize it so it's different every single time. You also never know what card you are going to get, so it's always a surprise!

To do this workout, all you need is a deck of cards, a big space free of obstacles, and some water. You will assign an exercise to each suit—diamonds, hearts, spades, and clubs. You can get creative here and assign all cardio-based moves, strength moves, moves for upper body, just lower body, or a combination. Really, whatever suits your goals goes!

The number of the card will be how many reps you do for each exercise. Personally, I like to call face cards and aces 10 reps. For example, if you draw a 3 of clubs, you will do 3 repetitions of whatever exercise you have assigned to clubs before continuing on to draw the next card. This is also a fun workout to do in a group!

I wanted to give you a full-body workout, so I've assigned the suits as such. However, feel free to assign the suits in a way that works for you. In terms of resting, you will be resting as needed, so no set rest periods. Just try to make them as short as possible and try to rest less from week to week.

In terms of timing, this workout will be most effective if done in around 15 minutes. However, newer exercisers may want to shorten this to 10 minutes and build up as their endurance and strength increase.

The Workout

HEARTS = BODYWEIGHT SQUATS

DIAMONDS = MOUNTAIN CLIMBERS

SPADES = PUSHUPS (KNEES ON THE GROUND OR LIFTED)

CLUBS = ALTERNATING SIDE LUNGES

Pick a card and do as many repetitions of the corresponding exercise as the number on the card. Draw another card and repeat for 15 minutes, resting as needed.

NOTES

Chapter 1: Embrace Imperfect Perfection
1. Gretchen Saffles, *Proverbs 31: Women of Dignity, Washed in Grace* (Lawrenceville, GA: Well-Watered Women Co., 2015), 68.
2. Ibid.

Chapter 2: Find Your Worth
1. As with all baking, please weigh your flour to ensure accurate results.

Chapter 5: Discover Your Roots
1. Gretchen Saffles, *Redefined Study: Defining Identity through the Mirror of God's Word* (Lawrenceville, GA: Well-Watered Women Co., 2017), 11.
2. Warren E. Berkley, "God's Work, God's Image, God's Distinction," The Expository Files (November 2002), accessed August 28, 2019, http://www.bible.ca/ef/expository-genesis-1-27; Steve Ham, "What Is the Image of God?" August 15, 2015, https://answersingenesis.org/genesis/what-is-image-of-god/.
3. Gary Michuta, "Adam and the Fig Leaf: An Uncomfortable Wardrobe Choice," Detroit Catholic, June 25, 2015, http://detroitcatholic.com/news/gary-michuta/adam-and -the-fig-leaf-an-uncomfortable-wardrobe-choice.
4. "What Is the Meaning of I AM WHO I AM in Exodus 3:14?" Got Questions Ministries, http://www.gotquestions.org/I-AM -WHO-I-AM-Exodus-3-14.html.

5. Saffles, *Redefined Study*, 22.

Chapter 6: Use Social Media for Good
1. John Piper, "Why Have You Made Me This Way?" Desiring God, July 21, 2015, https://www.desiringgod.org/labs/why-have-you-made-me-this-way.

Chapter 7: Feel the Fear and Do It Anyway
1. Christine Hebert, *The Eating with Grace Podcast*.

Chapter 8: Think about What Is True and Lovely
1. Joyce Meyer, *Battlefield of the Mind: Winning the Battle of Your Mind* (New York: Warner Faith, 2002).
2. Nicole Unice, *She's Got Issues: A DVD Group Experience* (Carol Stream, IL: Tyndale, 2013).
3. To do this, hold your kettlebell horizontally, so one hand is on each end. While holding it, squat low, and then jump up while pushing the kettlebell over your head like a shoulder press.

Chapter 9: Embrace the Almost but Not Yet
1. Beth Moore, *Breaking Free*, Updated Edition (Nashville: Lifeway, 2009), 11.

Chapter 10: Walk the Walk into Freedom
1. C. S. Lewis, *The Weight of Glory* (San Francisco: HarperOne, 2009), 26.
2. If you're dealing with hypothalamic amenorrhea, I strongly recommend reading the book *No Period. Now What?* by Nicola Rinaldi. It outlines the recovery process in detail, and it's the process I used to heal my body and mind.

Food *faith* Fitness

nourishing your body, mind and soul

Since you're reading this book, I imagine you're a woman who wants to approach health from a mentally and spiritually healthy way, and I have *just* the thing for you.

Introducing: my Body, Mind & Soul method!

This is my process for helping women restore their relationship with their bodies and get to a healthy weight while still fostering a mentally healthy relationship with food and Christ.

If that sounds like something you want, then I would love for you to download my free *Body, Mind & Soul Guide*, which will give you some of my best tips to make your body healthy, keep your mind on the right track, and keep your soul in alignment with Christ.

You'll learn the following:

- how to structure a meal to support your hunger and metabolic rate
- how to use journaling to renew your mind
- what it means to have a healthy soul, with tips to help you get there

Download this free guide here:

www.foodfaithfitness.com/bodymindsoul.

Or if you're a woman struggling with restriction and a lot of food "rules" (and maybe even a loss of your period, like me), then I would love to invite you to watch my free faith-based food freedom master class.

Watch the free training here:

www.foodfaithfitness.com/FFwebinar.